W. O. Seiler, H. B. Stähelin (Eds.) ■ **Malnutrition in the Elderly**

W. O. Seiler · H. B. Stähelin
Editors

Malnutrition in the Elderly

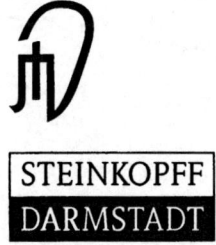

STEINKOPFF
DARMSTADT

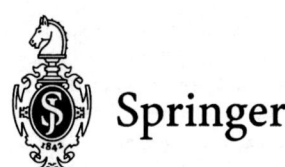

Springer

Editors' addresses:

Prof. Dr. med. W. O. Seiler
Prof. Dr. med. H. B. Stähelin
Geriatrische Universitätsklinik
Kantonsspital
CH-4031 Basel, Switzerland

Die Deutsche Bibliothek – CIP-Einheitsaufnahme

Malnutrition in the elderly / W. O. Seiler ; H. B. Stähelin (ed.) –
Darmstadt : Steinkopff, 1999
ISBN-13: 978-3-642-47075-2   e-ISBN-13: 978-3-642-47073-8
DOI: 10.1007/978-3-642-47073-8

Medical Editor: Beate Rühlemann – English Editor: Mary K. Gossen
Production: Heinz J. Schäfer
Cover Design: Erich Kirchner, Heidelberg
Typesetting: Typoservice, Griesheim
Printed on acid-free paper

Chronic diseases represent a high risk for inducing masked malnutrition. The number of acute and chronic diseases per patient is rapidly increasing with the growing number of elderly people leading to the known multimorbidity. At present, more than half of the ill elderly even in the industrialized world are suffering from malnutrition. Thus, the problems of malnurished elderly need more attention.

This book refers to the special aspects of malnutrition in the elderly and does not represent a comprehensive text book of dietetics. However, skilled international experts present in a precise manner methods for the early detection, prevention, and nutritional treatment of malnutrition.

This book should be especially appealing to nutrition educators, dietitians, geriatricians, and gerontologists. We trust that this book will prove useful to the interdisciplinary team members who bear the responsibility of caring for the frail elderly and of the nutritional education of the healthy elderly as well.

The editors and authors of this volume are grateful to the Novartis Foundation for Gerontological Research Basel for sponsoring the present book.

Basel, July 1999

W. O. SEILER
H. B. STäHELIN

Contents

Causes of malnutrition

Diagnosis of malnutrition

Treatment of malnutrition

Prevention of malnutrition

Introduction

H. B. Stähelin

"Under- or malnutrition is a frequent and serious problem in geriatric patients" (8). Today there is no doubt that malnutrition contributes significantly to morbidity and mortality in the aged. The immune function is impaired, the risk for falls and fractures increases, in acute illness, recovery is delayed, and complications are frequent. Acute and chronic illnesses lead to a catabolic metabolism and hence increase the signs and symptoms of malnutrition. Cytokines related to inflammation block the synthesis of albumin and shift protein synthesis to acute phase proteins. The activation of the ubiquitine-proteasome pathway leads to a degradation of muscle protein, which leads to an additional loss of muscle mass which occurs as age-dependent sarcopenia, and adds to the already existing frailty (2, 4). It is often difficult to decide to what extent the metabolic alterations result from malnutrition or concomitant illness.

Psychological factors contribute as a circulus vitiosus significantly to anorexia and, thus, aggravate the condition. They are the most important causes of failure to thrive in old age (7). It is evident that next to the therapy of the underlying illness, an adequate support with calorie and nutrient intake over weeks becomes essential under these conditions. Clear-cut improvements are often only seen after 6 or more weeks.

Besides a clinical, clearly visible malnutrition, selective nutrient deficits are much more frequent. Numerous and highly different mechanisms may lead to a marginal or insufficient supply with micronutrients. The clinical importance often remains unclear if the supply is in the low normal range. Long-lasting low supply with micronutrients correlates, however, in numerous studies with an increased incidence of chronic diseases.

In the animal experiment, a life-long caloric-restricted diet with sufficient supply of essential micronutrients diminishes morbidity and mortality and increases life expectancy (3). In humans, the strong interdependence of nutrient intake with a number of socio-economic and psychological factors which influence morbidity and mortality makes it difficult to prove a causal effect of calorie restriction on life expectancy. Nevertheless, overweight in young adult age is an important risk factor. In higher age, optimum life expectancy is associated with a slightly increased body mass index of 24–29 kg/m^2 (6). Elderly women exhibit in general a higher BMI than elderly men. This relates to a distinctly higher proportion of body fat. In the EURONUT-SENECA Study (9), over 30 % of the participants had a BMI of over 30 in 9 out of 19 study sites. At the same time, a significant number of persons were observed with a BMI value below 20 (in women up to 11 %). The high variance of BMI in women indicates that a number of medical, psychological, and social factors influence dietary intake in the older person. Therefore, the therapeutic approach in treating malnutrition has to be comprehensive. Not only the medical factors leading to a decreased nutrient intake, but also the psycho-social and economic influences have to be taken into account. Especially the physiological aging of taste and smell is underestimated and neglected. The insufficient stimulation of taste and smell contribute significantly to the frequently observed anhedonia and anorexia in the elderly. Thus, the increased avidity for sweets is rarely taken into account in preparing meals for the elderly (1, 5).

Nutrient deficits are frequent in the elderly. The mechanisms leading to these deficits are usually easily understood. However, the subtle changes are only detected if a careful and systematic search looks for signs and symptoms of malnutrition. Far too often, these findings are thought of as inevitable sequilae of illness or aging, and the genuine and causal importance of malnutrition is underestimated. It is the aim of this monograph to increase awareness of these interrelations and to demonstrate how by diagnosing and treating malnutrition, morbidity and mortality, as well as the cost of health care in the elderly can be significantly lowered, and quality of life improved.

References

1. DeCastro JM (1993) Age-related canges in spontaneous food intake and hunger in humans. Appetite 21: 255–272
2. Evans W (1997) Functional and metabolic consequences of sarcopenia. J Nutr 127 (Suppl 5): 998S–1003S
3. Finch CE (1990) Longevity, senescence, and the genome. University of Chicago Press. Chicago
4. Mitch WE, Goldberg AL (1996) Mechanisms of muscle wasting. The role of the ubiquitin-proteasome pathway. N Engl J Med 335: 1897–1905
5. Morley JE (1986) Nutritional status of the elderly. Am J Med 81: 679–695
6. National Research Council (1989) Diet and health. Implications for reducing chronic disease risk. National Academic Press. Washington DC, pp 563–592
7. Palmer RM (1990) Failure to thrive in the elderly: Diagnosis and management. Geriatrics 45 (9): 47–55
8. Schlierf G (1996) Mangelernährung geriatrischer Patienten. In: Ernährungsbericht 1996. Deutsche Gesellschaft für Ernährung (Hrsg). S. 233–250. DGE, Frankfurt
9. Seneca Investigators (1996) Longitudinal changes in anthropometric characteristics of elderly Europeans. Europ J Clin Nutr 50 (Suppl 2): S9–S15
10. Tucker HN, Miguel SG (1996) Cost containment through nutrition intervention. Nutr Reviews 54: 111–121

Author's address:

Prof. Dr. Hannes B. Stähelin
Geriatrische Universitätsklinik
Kantonsspital
CH-4031 Basel, Switzerland

Nutrient intake of healthy elderly subjects*
based on results of the SENECA Study "Nutrition and the elderly in Europe"

D. Schlettwein-Gsell[1], B. Decarli[2], J. A. Amorim Cruz[3], J. Haller[4],
C. P. G. M. de Groot[5], W. A. van Staveren[5]

1 Institute for Experimental Gerontology, Basel, Switzerland
2 Nestlé Research Center, Nestec Ltd, Lausanne, Switzerland
3 National Institute of Health, Lisbon, Portugal
4 Human Nutrition Research, F. Hoffmann-La Roche Ltd, Basel, Switzerland
5 Division of Human Nutrition and Epidemiology, Wageningen Agricultural University, Wageningen, The Netherlands

Summary

The SENECA study "Nutrition and the Elderly in Europe" is currently investigating men and women born 1913–1918 in 20 traditional small towns in Europe. At the age of 74–79 years subjective health was satisfactory or good in 95 % of 399 men and 93 % of 414 women in six study towns. In these subjects suboptimal blood levels of nutrients were virtually nonexistent. Food intake was low in energy and rich in protein and fat. Lowest European recommended dietary allowances of micronutrients were not reached by all subjects. Despite high nutrient density, the even higher amounts of vitamins and minerals recommended for their potentially protective effects were not reached by a substantial proportion of subjects with daily energy intakes of less than 6.3 MJ. Regularity of food intake was high and had increased over four years. Living alone did not adversely affect the quality of food intake, whereas low economic status did.

Introduction

Notwithstanding the confusingly large and ever-increasing number of publications on nutrition, relatively little is known about the actual diet of healthy elderly people. This is partly because much of the available data refers specifically to physically and/or mentally impaired elderly people living in institutions or sheltered accommodation and is therefore not applicable to the elderly population as a whole. An unbiased assessment is rendered even more difficult by the fact that in accordance with the social myth that elderly people are poor, ill, and lonely (11), studies on nutrition in the elderly often assume the diet of the elderly to be inadequate and

---

* This contribution was translated from German to English by David Playfair, 30 Cheverton Road, London N19 3AY, Great Britain, Email: DavidPlayfair@compuserve.com

therefore rarely undertake a search for positive aspects of the self-chosen diet of the elderly. It is therefore a welcome development that a longitudinal study that was started in 1988/9, the "SENECA Study Nutrition and the Elderly in Europe" (4, 5), is seeking to identify types of diet and living conditions that are associated with longevity and healthy aging. As this study is not due to end until 1999, no survival data are available at present. Nevertheless, it is possible on the basis of the results of the baseline study conducted in 1988/9 and the follow-up analysis of 1993 to characterize the dietary situation of healthy elderly people and to discuss the importance of certain risk factors.

Method and sample selection of the SENECA Study

The study, which is being coordinated by the Division of Human Nutrition and Epidemiology of Wageningen Agricultural University (CPGM de Groot, WA van Staveren, JGAJ Hautvast), is investigating a sample of men and women born 1913–1918 in 20 traditional small towns with a population of 10–20,000 inhabitants in 13 European countries. The highly standardized data collection comprises a questionnaire on way of life, a three-day recording of food intake, a dietary history based on a list of foods, anthropometric measurements, a Mini-Mental State Examination, a geriatric depression scale, a physical performance test, and a series of blood tests, most of which are performed in central laboratories. A first set of data collected in 1988/9 referred to 2590 subjects and a follow-up set collected in 1993 referred to 1431 subjects. Each of these sets of data has formed the basis of a publication (4, 5).

Nutritional status of healthy elderly subjects

In order to assess the nutritional status of healthy elderly subjects, the data from six SENECA towns in which more than 90 % of male and female subjects aged 74–79 years described their state of health as satisfactory or good were analyzed. These data refer to 399 men and 414 women from Hamme (Belgium), Roskilde (Denmark), Romans (France), Padua (Italy), Culemborg (Holland), and Yverdon (Switzerland).

From Table 1 it is apparent that the subjective state of health in these towns corresponds to objective criteria. The mean score in the Mini-Mental State Examination was over 27.2. Cognitive deficits are expected with scores of 23 or less (9). Only exceptionally were blood levels of vitamins, albumin, or haemoglobin suboptimal. In particular, plasma retinol (vitamin A) deficiency was nonexistent and suboptimal levels of α-tocopherol (vitamin E) or folic acid were present in less than 1.5 % of subjects. Especially noteworthy is the fact that mean levels of vitamin E and folic acid were found to have risen significantly since the baseline examination, which was conducted when the subjects were 70–75 years old (8). As compared with other studies, a relatively high proportion of subjects had serum cholesterol levels of less than 5.17 mmol/l (7).

Table 1. Nutritional state of healthy elderly men and women (born 1913–1918) from six SENECA study towns[a]. Follow-up study 1993 (5)

	Men	Women
	(n = 399)	(n = 414)
Percentage in whom subjective health satisfactory or good	95	93
	(n = 297)	(n = 299)
Mini-Mental State Examination[b] (score)	27.3	27.2
Percentage with suboptimal blood levels of vitamins[c]	(n = 343)	(n = 356)
Plasma retinol < 0.35 μmol/l	0	0
Plasma α-tocopherol < 11.6 μmol/l	1.5	0.3
α-tocopherol/cholesterol ratio < 2.5	0.6	0.3
Plasma vitamin B_{12} < 111 pmol/l	4.9	4.5
Plasma folic acid < 6.8 nmol/l	0	0.6
	(n = 101)	(n = 95)
Plasma vitamin B_6 < 20 nmol/l	2.0	3.1
	(n = 349)	(n = 357)
Serum albumin < 35 g/l	1.4	2.2
	(n = 349)	
Haemoglobin[d] < 126 g/l	2.9	
		(n = 351)
< 117 g/l		2.8
	(n = 354)	(n = 359)
Serum cholesterol < 5.16 mmol/l	28.6	14.2
> 6.45 mmol/l	20.3	41.8

[a] See "Method"; [b] No values for Hamme (Belgium); [c] Cut-off values for biochemical vitamin deficiency (8); [d] NHANES II criteria

Table 2. Percentage of healthy elderly men and women (born 1913–1918) from six SENECA study towns[a] with nutrient intakes below the lowest European recommendations[b]. Follow-up study 1993 (5)

	Men (n = 387)	Women (n = 405)
Percentage of subjects with:		
– energy intake < 6.3 MJ/day	8 (3–21)[c]	36 (17–55)[c]
– vitamin B_1 intake < 0.7 mg/day	24 (4–42)	29 (13–44)
– vitamin B_2 intake < 1.0 mg/day	28 (4–46)	20 (9–33)
– vitamin B_6 intake[d] < 0.8 mg/day	9 (4–17)	12 (6–20)
– vitamin C intake < 30 mg/day	4 (0–18)	6 (1–14)
– vitamin A intake < 600 RE/day	33 (3–83)	30 (4–81)
– calcium intake < 500 mg/day	10 (0–28)	13 (6–28)
– iron intake < 8 mg/day	10 (4–20)	17 (8–29)

[a] See "Method"; [b] Lowest European recommendation (RDA) (21); [c] Range of mean values in the individual towns; [d] No data for Padua (Italy). Men n = 318, women n = 339

Table 3. Nutrient density in healthy elderly men and women (born 1913–1918) from six SENECA study towns[a]. Follow-up study 1993 (5)

		Men (n = 387)	Women (n = 405)	Recommended density[b]
Vitamin B$_1$	mg/MJ	0.11 (0.09–0.13)[c]	0.12 (0.10–0.13)	0.14 mg/MJ
Vitamin B$_2$	mg/MJ	0.16 (0.12–0.20)	0.19 (0.14–0.21)	0.17 mg/MJ
Vitamin B$_6$[d]	mg/MJ	0.15 (0.13–0.17)	0.16 (0.14–0.18)	0.18 mg/MJ
Vitamin C	mg/MJ	9.3 (6.3 –12.7)	11.6 (8.3 –14.6)	8 mg/MJ
Vitamin A + β-carotene	RE/MJ	114 (59–185)	144 (73–217)	120 RE/MJ
Calcium	mg/MJ	100 (66–125)	116 (84–137)	110 mg/MJ
Iron	mg/MJ	1.4 (1.3–1.6)	1.5 (1.3–1.6)	1.4 mg/MJ

[a] See "Method"; [b] Nordic countriesí recommended nutrient densities for energy intake between 7 and 12.5 MJ (14); [c] Mean value of all subjects, range of mean values in individual towns; [d] No data for Padua (Italy). Men n = 318, women n = 339

The mean daily energy intake of the subjects in these towns was 7.9–10.4 MJ in men and 6.3–7.8 MJ in women, protein accounting for 14.9 % and 13.9 % respectively of the energy intake. The proportion of energy contributed by fat was 30–35 % in the southern towns and 40–44 % in the northern towns (13). From Table 2 it is also apparent that in all the towns considered a proportion of subjects did not consume the recommended dietary allowances of the various micronutrients (1). The dietary deficits of vitamin A were especially high. In some of the towns fewer than 20 % of subjects consumed the recommended amount of retinol. Despite this, no cases of biochemical vitamin A deficiency were found in any of the towns. As similar findings have been reported by other authors, it has for some time been conjectured that the vitamin A intake recommended for the elderly may be too high (17). Only minor dietary deficits with respect to recommendations were found for vitamin C and calcium, while rather larger deficits were found for the B-vitamins and iron.

As recommended intakes represent the mean physiological requirement plus two standard deviations and are thus adequate for 97 % of the population, few deficiencies are to be expected in a population even if up to a third of values lie below recommendations. It is therefore not surprising that the blood levels in the randomly selected elderly subjects of the SENECA study revealed no evidence of deficiency. Nevertheless, it is only thanks to high nutrient density (Table 3) that the intake of micronutrients required to prevent deficiency is achieved despite the relatively low energy consumption and total food consumption of these subjects. Avoidance of deficiencies also requires a knowledge of the value of individual foods. It is also important that elderly people cultivate the habit of routinely preparing nutritionally adequate meals even when their capacities diminish, their interest wanes, and they find themselves living alone.

The SENECA subjects are striking in terms of the routine and regularity of their food intake. Up to 90 % of subjects structured their midday and evening meals along the same pattern on all three study days (20). The proportion of subjects who had at least one hot meal each day was between 95 and 100 % overall, falling to 90 % only in the towns in which there is a tradition of not cooking on Saturdays (19).

The regularity of food intake increased over the four years of the study, a pattern already suspected on the basis of cross-sectional studies but previously undocumented (20) in longitudinal surreys. A lot of time and importance is given to meals. Most of the subjects spend between 30 and 60 minutes over the main meal of the day, while in some of the towns up to half the subjects spend more than an hour over their main meal (20).

Nevertheless, the supply of micronutrients needs to be assessed not only in terms of possible deficiencies, but also in terms of potential protective effects. This applies in particular to antioxidative substances. A vitamin E level of more than 30 µmol/l or a vitamin E/cholesterol ratio of more than 5.2 µmol/mmol is believed to provide protection against cardiovascular disease. In the SENECA follow-up study on subjects aged 74–79 years these values were 29 µmol/l and 5.6 µmol/mmol, respectively, in men and 33 µmol/l and 5.9 µmol/mmol, respectively, in women (8).

Subjects whose daily energy intake is less than 6.3 MJ are unlikely to be consuming protective amounts of micronutrients, though in subjects with such low energy intake the possibility of underreporting must always be borne in mind (22). Also, nutrient density was found to be higher in the subjects in the lowest than in those in the highest quartile of energy intake (2). Nevertheless, the elderly subjects whose energy intake is lowest do constitute a public health problem. An energy intake of less than 6.3 MJ/day is considered to be very unlikely to provide a qualitatively satisfactory diet. On the other hand, caloric restriction has been demonstrated to have beneficial effects on life expectancy and the development of chronic diseases in animals (12), and similar effects are conjectured in humans. It is therefore debatable whether an elderly person who feels well on a low-energy diet should be advised to eat more food. Elderly people often have only a limited ability to increase their energy requirements by undertaking more physical activity. Alternatively, the diet can be supplemented with nutrient-containing tablets. In the SENECA study, vitamin and mineral tablets were taken by 40–60 % of subjects in the northern European towns, 10–15 % of subjects in the central European towns, and less than 5 % of subjects in the southern European towns, however the use of these tablets was observed in the subjects with the lowest needs.

Risk factors for nutrition in the elderly

Living alone

Living alone is regularly listed as a risk factor in terms of a balanced diet in the elderly, though most studies on this question have failed to show this situation to have any negative influence on nutrient intake (15). In the SENECA study, 512 elderly subjects aged 70–75 years who lived alone in nine study towns were compared with 1397 subjects of the same age who did not live alone. An analysis of nutrient intake found the subjects who lived alone to have no nutritional deficits with respect to those who did not live alone. On the contrary, they consumed significantly larger amounts of vitamin A, riboflavin, and calcium, a phenomenon attributable to higher consumption of easily prepared milk products (15). These differences were independent of whether the subjects who lived alone were single, divorced, or recently or long-since widowed. Nor were the results influenced by the subjects' subjective health, economic problems, or isolation (expressed as "I don't know any of my neighbours") (19). As is true of people of all ages, the frequency of cooked meals was less and the number of meals eaten outside the home was greater in the elderly subjects of the SENECA study who lived alone than in those who did not (18). Nevertheless, over a period of 14 days 67 % of the men and 78 % of the women who lived alone ate all their meals alone at home. Asked whether they would prefer to have a cheap meal in a nearby club, 73 % of the women and 60 % of the men said that they preferred to have their meals at home (19). These findings contradict accepted socio-gerontological ideas to the effect that measures must be taken to improve the supposedly miserable and nutritionally unsatisfactory situation of elderly people who live alone. It seems that many of these "younger senior citizens" up to the age of 75 provide themselves with a balanced and nutritionally adequate diet despite living alone. It is not just in younger people that living alone is nowadays well regarded, and the ability to prepare one's own meals and the practice of actually doing so can be regarded as touchstones of this new autonomous way of life (10).

To what extent people beyond the age of 75 succeed in finding a satisfactory middle road between personal autonomy and new forms of dependence is not clear from the present data. It should not be forgotten that most cases of single status in the elderly arise out of loss of a partner and that this loss in itself may lead to social isolation.

Economic situation

Unlike living alone, economic situation is an important risk factor for quality of nutrition in the elderly. Those subjects of the SENECA study who reported difficulty in budgeting for their food purchases were found to have a significantly lower intake of three out of five nutrients analyzed than those subjects who reported no such difficulty. They were also almost four times as likely to describe their state of health as poor or very poor (19).

Thus, though it appears that elderly people up to the age of 75 who live alone and elderly people with minimal energy intake are able to overcome the difficulties that arise from these risk factors, economic difficulties are not so easily overcome. On the contrary, they lead – generally on a background of lifelong deficits in the realms of health, education, and social contacts – to a complex set of deprivations that cannot be overcome without external assistance.

Dentition

Defective dentition is likewise regarded as a nutritional risk factor in the elderly. Of 635 men and 718 women aged 74–79 years in the SENECA study, 3 % and 2 % respectively were edentulous without prostheses, 34 % and 46 % respectively were edentulous with full prostheses, 50 % and 43 % respectively had a combination of natural teeth and prostheses, and 13 % and 9 % respectively had natural teeth only. Difficulty in chewing was reported by 20 % of the men and 25 % of the women overall, was most common in the edentulous subjects without prostheses, and was more common in the subjects with a combination of natural teeth and prostheses than in those with full prostheses. Within the individual towns a number of interactions between dentition and nutrient intake were identified; however the only significant influence on nutrient intake to be found in the group of subjects as a whole was reduced intake of carbohydrates and vitamin B_6 in the few edentulous subjects without prostheses (6).

Favourite foods

The supposed preference of elderly people for soft, sweet foods – typified by pieces of bread dunked in milk coffee – is likewise regarded as a nutritional risk factor in old age. Around two thirds of the SENECA study subjects aged 74–79 years were able to nominate a food that they were particularly fond of eating. The favourite foods most frequently cited by the male subjects were traditional dishes (six towns), vegetables (three towns), and meat dishes in general (three towns), while those most frequently cited by the female subjects were vegetables (six towns) and meat dishes in general (four towns). Fruit was cited only rarely, namely by 0–3 % of the men in ten towns and by the same proportion of the women in six towns. This is a notable finding in view of the generally good intake of vitamin C in the subjects. In most of the towns the proportion of subjects citing sweets as their favourite food was very low, exceeding 10 % in only two towns in the case of men and four towns in the case of women. In an American comparative study, by contrast, 36 % of men and 24 % of women cited sweets as their favourite food (20). It is therefore not possible to make generalizations about "the favourite foods of the elderly".

Conclusions

On the basis of these findings it appears that within the limits of their capacities, healthy elderly people have an effective system for ensuring regular intake of food that they enjoy eating and that satisfies their physiological needs. This system, however, is extremely delicate. A minor disruption, an illness, an accident, a change of environment, or, far worse, the loss of someone close can drastically alter the diet and in combination with the reduced adaptability and resources of the elderly can lead to visible undernutrition within days. This clinical picture, which medical doctors often see in elderly people being admitted to hospital, has led to the assumption that elderly people in general have a poor diet (16).

The system is also delicate insofar as it is maintained by longstanding habits and regular consumption of high-quality food. Comparative regression analyses of food intake, hunger and stomach content suggest that with advancing age the motivation to eat comes to depend increasingly on external factors such as time of day, planned order of dishes, and social environment rather than on hunger or feelings of satiety (3). It is therefore important that the external environment that guarantees the elderly person's accustomed diet be kept intact. It is equally important that as they grow older, adults establish a firm habit of regular consumption of high-quality food.

References

1. Amorim Cruz JA, Moreiras O, Brzozowska A (1996) Longitudinal changes in the intake of vitamins and minerals of elderly Europeans. Eur J Clin Nutr 50 Suppl 2: 77–85
2. Barclay D, Decarli B, Dirren H, Schlettwein-Gsell D (1991) Dietary nutrient density and nutritional status of elderly with marginal energy intakes (abstract). First European Congress on Nutrition and Health, Nordwijkerhout Dec. 5–7
3. de Castro JM (1993) Age related changes in natural spontaneous food intake and hunger in humans. Appetite 22: 255–272
4. de Groot LCPGM, van Staveren WA, Hautvast JGAJ eds (1991) Euronut Seneca: Nutrition and the Elderly in Europe. Eur J Clin Nutr 45 suppl 3
5. de Groot LCPGM, van Staveren WA, Dirren H, Hautvast JGAJ eds (1996) Seneca: Nutrition and the Elderly in Europe, Follow-up study and longitudinal analysis. Eur J Clin Nutr 50 suppl 2
6. Fontijn-Tekamp FA, van't Hof MA, Slagter AP, van Waas MAJ (1996) The state of dentition in relation to nutrition in elderly Europeans in the SENECA study of 1993. Eur J Clin Nutr 50 suppl 2: 117–122
7. Grunenberger F, Lammi-Keefe CJ, Schlienger JL, Deslypere JP, Hautvast JGAJ (1996) Longitudinal changes in serum lipids of elderly Europeans. Eur J Clin Nutr 50 suppl 2: 25–31
8. Haller J, Weggemans RM, Lammi-Keefe CJ, Ferry M (1996) Changes in the vitamin status of elderly Europeans. Eur J Clin Nutr 50 suppl 2: 32–46
9. Haller J, Weggemans RM, Ferry M, Guigoz Y (1996) Mental health. Minimental state examination and geriatric depression score of elderly Europeans in the SENECA study of 1993. Eur J Clin Nutr 50 suppl 2: 112–116
10. Jaeggi E (1992) Ich sag mir selber guten Morgen – Single, eine moderne Lebensform. Munich, Piper
11. Lehr U (1974) Psychologie des Alters. Heidelberg, Quelle & Meyer
12. Masoro EJ (1992) Retardation of aging processes by food restriction. Am J Clin Nutr: 55 1250–1252
13. Moreiras O, van Staveren WA, Amorim Cruz JA, Carbagal A, de Henauw S, Grunenberger F, Roszkowski W (1996) Longitudinal changes in the intake of energy and macronutrients of elderly Europeans. Eur J Clin Nutr 50 suppl 2: 67–76
14. Nordisk Ministerrad (1989) Nordic nutrition recommendations, 2nd ed. PHUN Standing Committee on Food
15. Pearson JM, Schlettwein-Gsell D, van Staveren WA, de Groot LCPGM (1998) Living alone does not adversely affect nutrition intake and nutritional state of 70–75 year old men and women in small towns across Europe. Int J Food Sciences Nutrition 49: 131–139
16. Rapin CH, Feuz A, Weil R (1989) La malnutrition protéino-énergétique chez le malade âgé. Revue thérapeutique 46: 43–50
17. Russell RM, Suter PM (1993) Vitamin requirements of elderly people, an update. Am J Clin Nutr 58: 4–14
18. Schlettwein-Gsell D, Barclay D, Osler M, Trichopoulou A (1991) Dietary habits and attitudes. Eur J Clin Nutr 45 suppl 3: 83–96
19. Schlettwein-Gsell D, Barclay D (1995) Dietary habits and attitudes in healthy elderly. In Dall JLC et al (eds). Adaptations in Aging. London Academic Press 253–264

20. Schlettwein-Gsell D, Barclay D (1996) Longitudinal Changes in dietary habits and attitudes of elderly Europeans. Eur J Clin Nutr 50 suppl 2: 56–66
21. Trichopoulou A, Vassilakou T (1990) Recommended dietary intakes in Europe. Eur J Clin Nutr 44 suppl 2: 51–100
22. van Staveren WA, Burema J, Livingstone MBE, van den Brock T, Kaaks R (1996) Evaluation of the dietary history method used in the SENECA study. Eur J Clin Nutr 50 suppl 2: 47–55

Author's address:

Dr. D. Schlettwein-Gsell
Institute of experimental Gerontology
Socinstrasse 32
CH-4051 Basel, Switzerland

Nutritional status in ill elderly subjects*

W. O. Seiler

Geriatrische Universitätsklinik, Kantonsspital, Basel, Switzerland

Summary

Malnutrition in ill elderly subjects is one of the most common and at the same time least heeded problems in hospitals, nursing homes, and home care. Depending on the type and composition of the group of patients under consideration, the prevalence of malnutrition is cited at up to 60 %. The elderly eat considerably smaller amounts of food than the young and mostly eat food of low nutrient density. Especially at times of high energy requirements such as acute or chronic illness, this results in an energy deficit and general malnutrition. Precise diagnosis of malnutrition can be facilitated by determination of a number of biochemical parameters. Knowledge of these permits individualized nutritional therapy. The most important deficits affecting ill elderly subjects are those relating to proteins, iron, zinc, selenium, and vitamins B_{12}, B_1, B_6, and D. Malnutrition prolongs hospital stays, imposes enormous costs on health services, and causes considerable mortality. The present very rapid increase in the size of the elderly population will exacerbate the problem of malnutrition. More attention should therefore be paid to malnutrition by treating it as a disease in its own right and including it in the training of doctors and nurses.

Introduction

Malnutrition in ill elderly subjects is one of the most common and at the same time least heeded problems in hospitals, nursing homes, and home care (1, 17). It is certainly true to say that all chronically ill elderly patients show suboptimal nutritional parameters, i.e. suffer from malnutrition.

Whereas "only" 4–31 % of "healthy" elderly people living autonomously at home have subnormal nutritional parameters (16), up to 60 % of geriatric patients in acute hospital beds (18), long-term hospitals (9, 10), and nursing homes (23) show evidence of malnutrition (review by Abbasi & Rudmann (1)). The cited prevalence figures vary greatly because different criteria are used for the diagnosis of malnutrition and because patients in different studies are not homogeneous in terms

---

* This contribution was translated from German to English by David Playfair, 30 Cheverton Road, London N19 3AY, Great Britain, Email: DavidPlayfair@compuserve.com

Table 1. Biochemical parameters of nutrition

Proteins (acute and chronic-phase proteins)	Albumin, transferrin, ferritin, cholinesterase, prealbumin, retinol-binding protein
Lipids	Cholesterol, triglycerides
Minerals and trace elements	Sodium, potassium, magnesium, calcium, phosphorous, iron, selenium, zinc, copper
Vitamins	Vitamins B_{12}, B_1, and B_6, folic acid, vitamins C, D, and A
Other parameters	Absolute lymphocyte count, CD4/CD8 ratio, immunological skin tests

of morbidity. The greater the number of nutritional parameters determined, the greater is the likelihood of finding abnormal values.

As at present there are no generally accepted criteria for the diagnosis of malnutrition, the term malnutrition is defined here as the presence of one or more subnormal nutritional parameters. These include the biochemical parameters listed in Table 1 (6). It is also important to determine the severity of malnutrition. A proposed scheme for doing this is shown in Table 2.

The most important deficiency states affecting ill elderly subjects are discussed briefly below.

The most common deficiency states

Caloric deficiency

The elderly eat considerably smaller amounts of food, and eat less often, than the young. Especially at times of high energy requirements such as acute or chronic illness, this leads to an energy deficit and to general malnutrition (4). The principal reasons for this are: reduced energy requirement associated with reduced mobility; difficulties with eating, chewing, shopping, and preparation of meals; poverty; lack of movement; reduced muscular activity; age-related cytokine changes; and poor appetite as a result of gastrointestinal disorders or in many cases loneliness and depression. The fact that adequate nutrition requires a minimum caloric intake

Table 2. Severity of malnutrition (adapted from (17))

	Degrees of malnutrition			
	Normal	Mild	Moderate	Severe
Albumin (g/L)	45–35	35–32	31–28	< 28
Transferrin (g/L)	3.0–2.5	2.5–1.5	1.8–1.5	< 1.5
Prealbumin (mg/L)	300–150	150–120	120–100	< 100
Lymphocytes (/mm³)	5000–1500	1800–1500	1500–900	< 900
Serum zinc (μmol/L)	10.7–22.9	9.0–10.6	8.9–7.0	< 7.0

is often overlooked. Because their nutrient density is typically low, the meals eaten by the elderly are scarcely able to provide adequate amounts of nutrients. The elderly should be informed as early as possible of the importance of switching to foods of high nutrient density. Increased consumption of meat, dairy products, fish, eggs, and soya products should be aimed at (24).

Albumin deficiency

Hypoalbuminaemia is found in more than 60 % of malnourished geriatric patients. Albumin remains one of the most sensitive markers of malnutrition (17). Although albumin synthesis is reduced in favour of synthesis of acute-phase proteins in many conditions including acute and chronic infections, acute trauma, and burns, a low level of serum albumin should always be regarded as suggestive of malnutrition and should always trigger diagnostic measures to exclude malnutrition. Hypo-albuminaemia arises because diseases and multimorbidity in the elderly regularly result in the release of cytokines such as interleukin-1, interleukin-6, and TNF-alpha (5). These initiate a catabolic phase characterized by breakdown of muscle cells and rapid loss of appetite. The aversion of ill elderly people to meat is well known. Illness and lack of appetite maintain the catabolic state. This is a common situation in geriatric patients. As a result of lack of appetite and a specific cytokine pattern (5), food consumption falls. The situation is harmful in that it has two causes. In the first place, the disease leads to the catabolic state and the specific cytokine pattern seen also in acutely ill but still well-nourished younger patients in burns units or acute surgical wards (12). In chronically ill elderly patients the catabolism is compounded by a severe nutritional deficit that was generally present even before the patient's admission to hospital. This nutritional deficit arises because elderly people generally fall ill gradually the therefore – because of the resulting lack of appetite, aversion to meat, and reduced energy requirement – eat less than they usually do for some time before being admitted to hospital (4). It is for this reason that more than 60 % of ill elderly subjects already have an albumin deficit before or at the time that their metabolism switches over to a catabolic state because of acute illness (13). As this albumin deficit is scarcely noticed or is attributed to preexisting malnutrition (21), the malnutrition persists and may even become worse after the patient is admitted to hospital (1). Without prompt diagnosis and appropriate countermeasures the patient's nutritional parameters will deteriorate further from day to day. In this situation renutrition to restore normal nutritional parameters can take weeks or months.

Albumin deficiency impairs the immune response of the elderly (14). Protein-energy malnutrition is accompanied by a reduction in lymphocyte proliferation and cytokine production and impairs antibody response after vaccinations. Aging and malnutrition exert a cumulative negative effect on the immune response. For this reason even healthy elderly subjects, but far more so ill elderly subjects, are at increased risk of infection. Deficiencies of micronutrients and vitamins, which always accompany protein-calorie malnutrition, have a profound effect on the immune system (8). Malnutrition must be promptly identified and treated in order to reduce the risk of infection and possibly to retard the processes of aging.

Vitamin B$_{12}$ deficiency

At about 40 %, the prevalence of vitamin B$_{12}$ deficiency in ill elderly subjects is much greater than that in younger subjects. This deficiency is partly nutritional, i.e. due to inadequate intake of the vitamin in food. In addition, however, there is mounting evidence that cobalamin malabsorption increases with age, probably as a result of autoimmune atrophic gastritis (2, 19). The principal manifestations of cobalamin deficiency in the elderly are peripheral neuropathy and reduced nerve conduction velocity (20), reversible psychiatric illnesses, in particular delirium, and cognitive disturbances including dementia (3, 22). Slight macrocytosis is often present, but macrocytic anaemia is relatively rare. The presence of macrocytosis in an elderly subject is therefore not a reliable diagnostic indicator of vitamin B$_{12}$ deficiency, a circumstance that to a considerable extent explains why the diagnosis of vitamin B$_{12}$ deficiency in the elderly is so often missed. This diagnosis must be considered long before the appearance of marked macrocytosis or anaemia. Cobalamin replacement therapy is cheap and harmless, and if started early enough can prevent the development of these conditions. As the vitamin B$_{12}$ storage capacity of the liver of the elderly is not five years, as in younger people, but in many cases only a few months, replacement therapy must be given several times per year. Moreover, the normal range of serum vitamin B$_{12}$ level cited in reference tables is far too low. In fact, serum levels in the lower part of the traditional normal range of 125–320 µmol/L are indicative of an inadequate supply of vitamin B$_{12}$ (19). In such cases the diagnosis of vitamin B$_{12}$ deficiency can be confirmed by determination of serum levels of methylmalonate and homocysteine or response to vitamin B$_{12}$ replacement. Atrophic gastritis can be diagnosed indirectly by determination of serum levels of gastrin and pepsinogen. Atrophic gastritis results in malabsorption of protein-bound cobalamin present in food. Under these conditions the Schilling test, which uses unbound cobalamin, is uninformative (2). In severe malnutrition and vitamin B$_{12}$ deficiency the need for gastroscopy should also be considered.

The elderly respond well to vitamin B$_{12}$ therapy in terms of macrocytosis, anaemia, and neuropathy. Once severe dementia is present, however, no improvement in cognitive functions can be expected, though the risk of delirium is reduced by treatment.

Risk factors for cobalamin deficiency are atrophic gastritis, a history of partial gastrectomy, autoimmune diseases such as insulin-dependent diabetes mellitus and disorders of thyroid function, and long-term therapy with potent modern inhibitors of gastric acid secretion.

The relative contributions of inadequate nutrition and malabsorption to the unexpectedly high prevalence of vitamin B$_{12}$ deficiency and the even more common finding of marginal vitamin B$_{12}$ status in the elderly are not yet fully know. Current large-scale intervention studies on vitamin B$_{12}$, folic acid, and pyridoxine (vitamin B$_6$) may elucidate this question and lead to changes in the normal ranges of the serum levels of these vitamins.

Trace elements

Serum levels of the micronutrients iron and zinc are reduced in up to 60 % of geriatric patients (13).

Serum iron is often low in chronic infections, antirheumatic drug therapy, gastrointestinal diseases, and multimorbidity, whereas except under conditions of considerable stress, low serum zinc is indicative of protein malnutrition. Zinc is therefore regarded as a good indicator of nutritional status. The principal causes of zinc deficiency in the elderly are a meat-free diet and inadequate food intake. Given the generally small amounts of food eaten by the elderly, only dairy products and meat of very high nutrient density have zinc concentrations sufficient to ensure adequate intake of this trace element.

Zinc is a constituent of over a hundred enzymes, including in particular transcription enzymes, which play a critical role in protein synthesis. Zinc deficiency halts hepatic albumin synthesis, retards wound healing, and impairs immune response (7). By reducing appetite and causing dysgeusia, zinc deficiency sets up a vicious circle that maintains malnutrition (15). Severe malnutrition, which in the elderly is always accompanied by zinc deficiency, requires zinc replacement therapy, as even after food intake has returned to normal the small amounts of zinc present in normal food are insufficient to re-establish the depleted stores of zinc in the muscles and liver. The body's zinc stores last only a few weeks unless replenished by zinc ingested with food. Zinc deficiency is therefore an early indicator of incipient malnutrition. Organic zinc compounds are the best absorbed form of zinc for replacement therapy. Once all nutritional parameters have returned to normal, no further zinc replacement therapy is required (11, 14).

Conclusion

Elderly subjects always have inadequate nutritional parameters after a few weeks of illness. Malnutrition is therefore the most common comorbid condition of the elderly. Notwithstanding this, scant attention is paid to it because it does not yet form part of the training of doctors and nurses (17). Planned changes in medical courses should take account of demographic shifts, in particular the current very rapid increase in the size of the elderly population, by including the diseases likely to be suffered by the future population in the medical curriculum.

References

1. Abbasi AA, Rudman D (1994) Undernutrition in the nursing home: prevalence, consequences, causes and prevention. Nutr Rev 52: 113-122
2. Aimone-Gastin I, Pierson H, Jeandel C, Bronowicki JP, Plenat F, Lambert D, Nabet-Belleville F, Gueant JL (1997) Prospective evaluation of protein bound vitamin B_{12} (cobalamin) malabsorption in the elderly using trout flesh labelled in vivo with ^{57}Co-cobalamin. Gut 41: 475-479
3. Assantachai P, Yamwong P, Chongsuphaijaisiddhi T (1997) Relationships of vitamin B_1, B_{12}, folate and the cognitive ability of the Thai rural elderly. J Med Assoc Thai 80: 700-705
4. Blumberg J (1997) Nutritional needs of seniors. J Am Coll Nutr 16: 517-523
5. Bonnefoy M, Coulon L, Bienvenu J, Boisson RC, Rys L (1995) Implication of cytokines in the aggravation of malnutrition and hypercatabolism in elderly patients with severe pressure sores. Age-Ageing 24: 37-42
6. Braunwald E, Isselbacher KJ, Petersdarf RG, Wilson JD, Martin JB, Fauci AS (1987) Harrison's Principles of Internal Medicine. McGraw-Hill, New York

7. Buzina-Suboticanec K, Buzina R, Stavljenic A, Farley TM, Haller J, Bergman-Markovic B, Gorajscan M (1998) Ageing, nutritional status and immune response. Int J Vitam Nutr Res 68: 133–141

8. Chandra RK (1997) Nutrition and the immune system: an introduction. Am J Clin Nutr 66: 460S– 463S

9. Gilmore SA, Robinson G, Posthauer ME, Raymond J (1995) Clinical indicators associated with unintentional weight loss and pressure ulcers in elderly residents of nursing facilities. J Am Diet Assoc 95: 984–992

10. Giner M, Laviano A, Meguid MM, Gleason JR (1996) In 1995 a correlation between malnutrition and poor outcome in critically ill patients still exists (see comments). Nutrition 12: 23–29

11. Girodon F, Lombard M, Galan P, Brunet-Lecomte P, Monget AL, Arnaud J, Preziosi P, Hercberg S (1997) Effect of micronutrient supplementation on infection in institutionalized elderly subjects: a controlled trial. Ann Nutr Metab 41: 98–107

12. Hill AA, Plank LD, Finn PJ, Whalley GA, Sharpe N, Clark MA, Hill GL (1997) Massive nitrogen loss in critical surgical illness: effect on cardiac mass and function. Ann Surg 226: 191–197

13. Lauber C (1994) Bedeutung von Zink bei geriatrischen Patienten und Interpretation des Serum-Zink-Spiegels als Ernährungsparameter. Thesis, Medical Faculty, University of Basel

14. Lesourd BM (1997) Nutrition and immunity in the elderly: modification of immune responses with nutritional treatments. Am J Clin Nutr 66: 478S–484S

15. Mahajan SK, Prasad AS, Lambujon J, Abbasi AA, Briggs WA, McDonald FD (1980) Improvement of uremic hypogeusia by zinc: a double-blind study. Am J Clin Nutr 33: 1517–1521

16. McCormack P (1997) Undernutrition in the elderly population living at home in the community: a review of the literature. J Adv Nurs 26: 856–863

17. Morley JE, Glick Z, Rubenstein LZ (1995) Geriatric nutrition: a comprehensive review. Raven Press, New York

18. Naber TH, Schermer T, de Bree A, Nusteling K, Eggink L, Kruimel JW, Bakkeren J, van Heereveld H, Katan MB (1997) Prevalence of malnutrition in nonsurgical hospitalized patients and its association with disease complications (see comments). Am J Clin Nutr 66: 1232–1239

19. Nilsson-Ehle H (1998) Age-related changes in cobalamin (vitamin B_{12}) handling. Implications for therapy. Drugs Aging 12: 277–292

20. Oishi M, Mochizuki Y (1998) Improvement of P300 latency by treatment of vitamin B_{12} deficiency. J Clin Neurophysiol 15: 173–174

21. Pokrywka HS, Koffler KH, Remsburg R, Bennett RG, Roth J, Tayback M, Wright JE (1997) Accuracy of patient care staff in estimating and documenting meal intake of nursing home residents. J Am Geriatr Soc 45: 1223–1227

22. Rabins P (1998) Pernicious anemia and reversible dementia: Strachan and Henderson 30 years later. Int J Geriatr Psychiatry 13: 139–140

23. Rudman D, Abbasi AA, Isaacson K, Karpiuk E (1995) Observations on the nutrient intakes of eating-dependent nursing home residents: underutilization of micronutrient supplements (see comments). J Am Coll Nutr 14: 604–613

24. Sullivan D, Lipschitz D (1997) Evaluating and treating nutritional problems in older patients. Clin Geriatr Med 13: 753–768

Autor's address:

Prof. Dr. med. Walter O. Seiler
Geriatrische Universitätsklinik
Kantonsspital
CH-4031 Basel, Switzerland

Physiopathology of the catabolism associated with malnutrition in the elderly

D. Baez-Franceschi, J. E. Morley[1]

University of Puerto Rico Medical Sciences Campus, Internal Medicine Department, Geriatric Medicine Section, San Juan, PR; [1] Dammert Professor of Gerontology, Saint Louis University Health Sciences Center, Division of Geriatric Medicine, St. Louis, MO, USA

Summary

Malnutrition is a very common condition in the aging population. The reasons for this are multiple ranging from socio-economical factors to physiologic and pathologic alterations associated to growing old. Multiple changes related to the aging process in feeding modulators for instance, cholecystokinin, opioids, leptin, and nitric oxide are described in the scientific literature and are reviewed. Cytokines, their role in feeding behavior, and the alterations in their effects in the elderly are also studied. The interplay of these neurotransmitters, hormones, and cytokines is evaluated to examine why older persons might be at a higher risk of developing malnutrition. The association of cytokines with catabolism, and anorexia is also discussed.

Introduction

Malnutrition is a common finding amongst our elders (14). The causes of malnutrition are multifactorial and although they have been extensively studied, they are not entirely understood. Both physiological and pathological processes of aging put this population at a higher risk of being undernourished. These may be related to social, financial, psychological and/or physiological changes directly or indirectly associated to growing old.

Physiological alterations resulting from the normal course of aging have been linked with augmented probability of developing a poor nutritional status. A recent comparative study between young and older individuals found that after having a solid meal, aged subjects had less desire to eat, reduced hunger and slower gastric emptying for both solids and liquids when compared to their younger counterparts (9). Other alterations in the physiology of older people have been found to affect feeding behavior in this population. To better understand the pathophysiology of appetite regulation, we will review what is known concerning appetite regulation, and then discuss which factors are altered during normal aging. Finally, we will address the catabolic metabolism associated with malnutrition in some of the aged.

Factors controlling feeding drive

The feeding drive is regulated by multiple systems interacting with each other. Various tastes, odors, and even chewing quality may affect appetite. In addition, there are peripheral satiety messages from both the gut and fat cells that interact with a central feeding system. Within the central nervous system, the paraventricular nucleus, ventromedial nucleus, arcuate nucleus, and the lateral hypothalamus are affected by different stimuli that range from neuropeptides and hormones to cytokines.

In the late 1970s cholecystokinin (CCK) was recognized as playing a role in the satiation produced after a meal in rodents (64). Since these pioneering studies, multiple gastrointestinal hormones, such as amylin, gastrin-releasing peptide, glucagon, glucagon-like peptide, and somatostatin, have been shown to decrease food intake in animals and humans (4, 8, 20, 29, 32, 39, 50, 52, 56). Several of these appear to produce their effect by stimulating ascending fibers in the vagus. Adipose cells produce leptin, another hormone that decreases appetite (65). Within the central nervous system monoamines (norepinephrine, serotonin), peptides (dynorphin, neuropeptide Y, corticotrophin releasing hormone, and the orexins) and nitric oxide modulate food intake (5, 13, 33, 37, 38, 43, 51, 60, 62). It is the interplay of these multiple neurotransmitters and hormones that ultimately make the organism decide to seek food.

Age related anorexia

Age associated changes increase the risk of malnutrition in older individuals. These alterations range from problems in taste and smell perception, which were previously thought to be the main cause of anorexia in this population, to alterations in either the concentration or efficacy of the previously mentioned feeding modulators.

After an overnight fast, elderly subjects have less hunger and desire to eat than their younger counterparts (10). Following a meal, older subjects have less desire to eat and hunger, although the fullness sensation was not different when compared to young people. In this same study in elderly persons, gastric emptying was slower for both solids and liquids.

Many studies in animal models demonstrate changes in hormones and neurotransmitters at different levels that may be responsible for the differences that occur with aging. Cholecystokinin's concentration has been found to be three times as high in the duodenal mucosa of aged guinea pigs together with a higher receptor affinity that could be related to a stronger satiety effect postprandially. Human studies have also found elevated cholecystokinin levels in older persons, though this may be associated with malnutrition (46). Pancreatic receptors for cholecystokinin decrease in number, which may be associated with the malabsorption commonly seen in the elderly (59). Cholecystokinin has also been found to be more anorectic in aged rodents (66, 71).

Opioids (especially the kappa agonist, e.g., dynorphin) show a progressive decline with aging in mice (35). This reduced sensitivity to opioids with increasing age was also observed in rats treated with naloxone, a potent opioid antagonist (25). Opioid receptors in the brain also decline with increasing age (53).

Leptin mRNA is directly associated with adipose tissue, plasma glucose, and insulin levels in all age groups (47). Leptin levels also correlate with body fat in healthy female elders, but in chronically ill older adults, leptin was found to be low and had no relation to body fat; thus, other factors must be involved in the malnutrition of chronic disease (7). In older human females, leptin levels decline with age, in concert, with the loss of total adipose tissue. In older males, there is an interaction between testosterone and body fat in determining leptin levels. Testosterone inhibits leptin (3), and as with aging there is a decline in testosterone levels (55) there tends to be a relatively higher leptin level for a given quantity of fat in males. Thus, leptin may play a role in the regulation of anorexia in older males.

A recently discovered modulator of food intake is nitric oxide (NO), which enhances appetite. When a NO antagonist was administered to mice of different ages, older animals had higher sensitivity to its effect producing more anorexia in this group (54). Besides, a direct effect of NO within the hypothalamus, NO is responsible for adaptive relaxation of the fundus of the stomach. Early satiation in older persons appears to be due, in part, to failure of the fundus to display adequate adaptive relaxation.

Increased intestinal malabsorption is very common in the elderly population and may account in part for the malnutrition observed in this group. Although older mice have the same intestinal adaptive mechanisms as young ones, there is impairment on the ability to regulate nutrient uptake when older mice are given dietary challenges (19). The pancreatic exocrine response to different diets is also affected with aging, further contributing to subclinical malabsorption (26).

Although not directly caused by the aging process, several conditions may directly effect the nutritional status of an already compromised person. These include chronic inflammatory states, acute infectious processes, injuries, neoplasms, and chronic diseases. Cytokines play a leading role in the pathophysiology of malnutrition in these situations.

Anorexia and cytokines

Several conditions such as anorexia nervosa, cancer, infectious conditions, and inflammatory processes are associated with decreased food intake and weight loss. These conditions present with elevated levels of immunoregulatory substances known as cytokines. Each of these cytokines has multiple effects (Fig. 1).

Interleukin-1 (IL-1), which increases in infectious processes, inflammatory arthritis, and neoplasias, is partially responsible for the anorexia and weight loss seen in these illnesses. The mechanism by which IL-1 exerts these effects involves several pathways. IL-1 along with tumor necrosis factor (TNF) and endotoxin directly stimulate the expression of leptin mRNA in hamsters (27). This effect of IL-1 (and also, of TNF and lipopolysaccharide (LPS) of elevating leptin levels was also observed after intraperitoneal injection in mice (63). In humans with cancer, intravenous (IV) administration of IL-1 alpha also stimulates the production of leptin and causes anorexia (34). In addition to its effect on leptin levels, IL-1 also

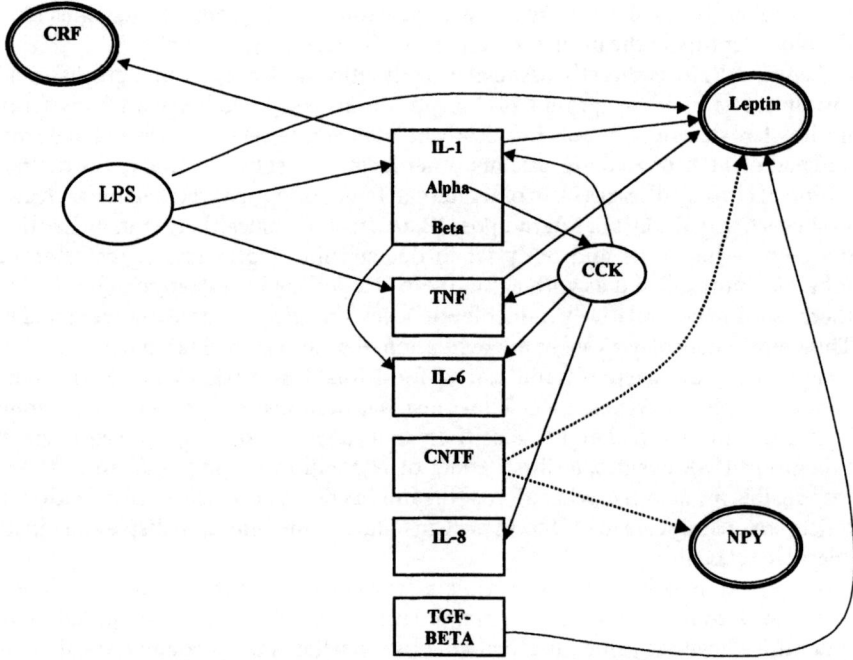

Fig. 1. Cytokines and their interaction with neurotransmitters and hormones associated with modulation of food intake; ——▶ : excitatory stimuli; ---▶ : inhibitory stimuli.

induces interleukin 6 (IL-6), which is associated with decreasing food intake and is involved in the acute-phase response (24, 57). Chronic intracerebroventricular infusion of IL-1 beta caused anorexia and increased levels of IL-6 in rats without evidence of the tachyphylaxis observed with IL-1 alpha (21). Corticotrophin-releasing factor (CRF) also mediates to some extent the suppression of food intake. IL-1 directly stimulated CRF's secretion from the hypothalamus (70). Furthermore, interleukin-1 alpha injection increased CCK plasma levels in rats. Following CCK antagonist treatment, the IL-1 alpha effect that provoked anorexia and delayed gastric emptying was partially blocked (12), demonstrating another method by which IL-1 may render its actions. In vitro studies of monocytes from healthy human subjects stimulated with CCK showed increased levels of IL-1, TNF, IL-6, and IL-8; all of which have been associated with a synergistic decrease in food intake after intracerebroventricular administration in rats (11, 68).

Tumor necrosis factor acts synergistically with IL-1 to produce anorexia in rats, and both develop tolerance to chronic intravenous infusion (74). The effect of TNF- alpha apart from being synergistic is additive when administered with IL-1 beta intracerebroventricularly in lean and obese rats (58). Intracerebroventricular injection of TNF-alpha also reduces food intake in pigs and increases cortisol levels (72).

TGF-beta enhances the expression of ob-mRNA in mouse adipocytes increasing leptin levels, which could be one of the pathways leading to anorexia in persons under an acute stress such as inflammation or an overwhelming infection (28). However, in the same study a decrease in ob-mRNA expression was observed when these adipocytes were stimulated with IL-1 beta, IL-6, IL-11, and TNF-alpha which contrasts with the above mentioned findings. The starvation seen in anorexia nervosa is also associated with increased serum levels of TGF-beta and IL-6.

Ciliary neurotrophic factor (CNTF) is part of the IL-6 family of cytokines. When CNTF is given as an intracerebroventricular infusion to rats, it is associated with decreased levels of NPY gene expression and anorexia. Nevertheless, CNTF also decreases leptin mRNA in lipocytes, so most probably leptin is not involved in the feeding suppression caused by this cytokine (73). CNTF also potentiates the production of corticosterone and IL-6 induced by IL-1 (17).

Cytokines and aging

After discussing the effects of the different cytokines on feeding behavior, we will now explore how the aging process affects them.

In 1990, a study done in humans revealed no association among cytokines and aging or even weight loss. Blood samples of healthy young, healthy elderly, chronically ill elderly, and nursing home individuals were evaluated for basal levels of TNF and IL-1. They were then correlated with age and weight loss. No statistical differences were found among the groups (48).

Despite the fact that no difference in basal concentrations of cytokines have been observed among young and old persons, the levels of TNF, IL-1, and others do rise after stimulation. Intracerebroventricular infusion of lipopolysaccharide to old rats did not alter monocyte counts when compared with young rats. Nevertheless, TNF levels in the cerebrospinal fluid of these older rodents were markedly increased (67). These findings suggest that cells from aged subjects may have a greater capacity to produce some of the cytokines.

Another study comparing children's and adults' production of cytokines found that the levels of interleukin-2 (IL-2), interleukin-4 (IL-4), IL-6, and interferon-gamma (Ifn-gamma) were higher in young adults after mitogen stimulation (40). Healthy elderly persons increased their production of IL-6, TNF-alpha, and IL-1 beta following stimulation with mitogens when compared to young healthy subjects (16). Cytokine antagonists' concentrations are also augmented in apparently healthy older adults (6). Since this was associated to a higher neopterin concentration, which is a marker of cell mediated immunity, it could be hypothesized that healthy elderly subjects may have subclinical chronic monocyte activation resulting in higher levels of circulating cytokines.

Besides the increasing production of TNF with aging, a recent report indicated that TNF produced in adipose tissue of older rodents is more active than that of young animals (49). Thus, we can speculate that TNF's actions on feeding behavior may also be stronger in elderly persons.

On the other hand, cancer patientís levels of IL-1, IL-6, and TNF-alpha did not correlate with anorexia or weight loss in subjects whose age ranged from 26–92 years (44). This means that we still do not know the complete story of how anorexia, aging, and all of its causes interact, and more research needs to be done.

Cytokines and catabolism

Besides from their association with decreased food intake, cytokines are also related to increased muscle protein breakdown during severe infectious processes, injuries, and neoplasias. We will explore their role in the catabolic metabolism that occurs in some cases of malnutrition in the elderly.

Tumor necrosis factor-alpha increased muscle protein breakdown in rats, decreased liver proteolysis, and when IL-1 is added to TNF infusion, it acted synergistically to produce these effects (22). In rats receiving intraperitoneal TNF, urine nitrogen excretion increased, there was a significant reduction of heart and liver protein content, and 3-methylhistidine, an indicator of muscle protein breakdown, was also augmented although its increased level did not reach statistical significance (42). In vitro activity of TNF on human adipose tissue inhibits lipo-protein lipase activity, preventing the hydrolysis of triglycerides to free fatty acids in the blood and, thus, impeding their storage in adipose tissue (23).

Female mice infected with cysts of Toxoplasma gondii are hypermetabolic, anorexic, and have weight loss accompanied by increased levels of IL-1, IL-2, IL-4, IL-5, IL-6, IL-10, Ifn-gamma, and TNF in the acute phase of the infection (1). In the chronic phase, the surviving mice that were still hypermetabolic and anorectic still had elevated levels of all the above mentioned cytokines, in particular: IL-4, IL-5, IL-10, and IL-6. Intravenous infusion of TNF and IL-1 caused weight loss, decreased food intake, net nitrogen loss, skeletal muscle catabolism, and increased liver weight in rats. TNF had a greater effect on muscle protein catabolism, due to a slight decrease in protein synthesis and a slight increase in breakdown, and on liver weight gain caused by liver protein anabolism. IL-1 was associated with tachy-phylaxis (41).

Chronic intracerebroventricular infusion of IL-1 in rats besides reducing body weight and food intake in rats, also elevates body temperature and produces significant nitrogen loss. In addition, IL-1 increased adrenal weight and corticosterone levels (31). Since glucocorticoids increase proteolysis of muscle, this is yet another possible pathway of catabolism. Contrary to TNF, IL-1 does not induce lipolysis; on the contrary, it is associated with increase synthesis of hepatic free fatty acids (18).

CNTF injected subcutaneously in female mice caused increase protein degradation besides increasing the acute phase reaction (15). It was also associated with development of muscle atrophy and weight loss when compared with pair fed animals. These effects were independent of TNF or IL-1 (45).

Conclusion

Cytokines play an important role in development of malnutrition. Not only do they have a direct effect on feeding modulators such as leptin, NPY, and CRF (Fig. 1); but there is evidence that following different stimuli, mononuclear cells produce higher

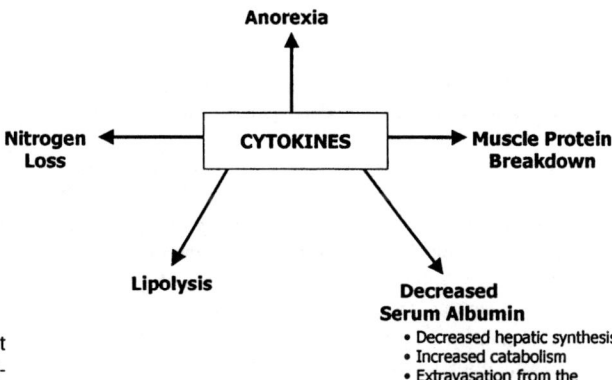

Fig. 2. Effects of cytokines that lead to weight loss and malnutrition.

concentrations of L-1 beta, IL-6, and TNF in older subjects. All of these are associated with decreasing food intake in animals and humans. Furthermore, one of the studies indicated that adipose tissue TNF increased its potency with increasing age. Since one of the effects of TNF is anorexia, it can be hypothesized that it may be more anorectic in older individuals.

There are multiple alterations of feeding regulators associated with aging, such as higher cholecystokinin concentration, a gradual decrease in sensitivity of the ability of opioids to induce food intake, higher leptin levels (in males), and greater sensitivity to NO inhibitors, among others. All of these, place even the successfully aged person in a precarious position when situations such as sepsis, chronic or acute inflammatory conditions, and cancer (which elevate cytokines) arise (30, 61, 69). This may be because some of the same cytokines that produce anorexia, also increase muscle protein breakdown, net nitrogen loss, lipolysis, and increase circulating levels of glucocorticoids (which have also been associated with proteolysis (36)) (Fig. 2). The sum of these can then be catastrophic, since it can lead to net metabolic catabolism.

There is another entity named by some as failure to thrive and more recently as senile or age-related anorexia. This condition is characterized by weight loss in elderly persons without an apparent cause. In 1994, elderly patients with idiopathic anorexia were compared with healthy older adults and healthy young people. Anorectic older patients showed significantly higher concentrations of IL-6 and TNF (2). Younger persons with anorexia nervosa also have higher levels of IL-6. Whether the cytokines are the cause of the syndrome or it is the anorexia per se which causes the cytokines be increased remains to be investigated. We can speculate that even if cytokines are not the principal mediators, they are involved in the cycle of anorexia and weight loss.

Finally, there is still much to be learned about appetite regulation. The role and actions of cytokines in the etiology of anorexia and catabolism are far from completely understood. Research directed to elucidate cytokine actions and their interplay with hormones, and neurotransmitters must continue to develop new and more effective therapies for these conditions.

References

1. Arsenijevic D, Girardier L, Seydoux J et al. (1997) Altered energy balance and cytokine gene expression in a murine model of chronic infection with Toxoplasma gondii. Am J Physiol 272: E908–E917

2. Arnalich F, Hernanz A, Vazquez JJ et al. (1994) Cell-mediated immune response and cytokine production in idiopathic senile anorexia. Mech Ageing Dev 77: 67–74

3. Behre HM, Simoni M, Nieschlag E (1997) Strong association between serum levels of leptin and testosterone in men. Clinical Endocrinology 47: 237–240

4. Bellinger LL, Williams FE (1986) Glucagon and epinephrine suppression of food intake in liver denervated rats. Am J Physiol 251: R349–R358

5. Billington CJ, Briggs JE, Grace M et al. (1991) Effects of intracerebroventricular injection of neuropeptide Y on energy metabolism. Am J Physiol 260: R321–R327

6. Catania A, Airaghi L, Motta P et al. (1997) Cytokine antagonists in aged subjects and their relation with cellular immunity. J Gerontol: Biological Sciences 52A: B93–B97

7. Cederholm T, Arner P, Palmblad J (1997) Low circulating leptin levels in protein-energy malnourished chronically ill elderly subjects. J Intern Med 242: 377–382

8. Chance WT, Balasubramaniam A, Stallion A et al. (1993) Anorexia following the systemic injection of amylin. Brain Res 607: 185–188

9. Clarkston WK, Pantano MM, Morley JE et al. (1997) Evidence for the anorexia of aging: Gastrointestinal transit and hunger in healthy elderly vs young adults. Am J Physiol 272: R243–R248

10. Cook CG, Andrews JM, Jones KL et al. (1997) Effects of small intestinal nutrient infusion on appetite and pyloric motility are modified by age. Am J Physiol 273: R755–R761

11. Cunninham ME, Shaw-Stiffel TA, Bernstein LH et al. (1995) Cholecystokinin stimulated monocytes produce inflammatory cytokines and eicosanoids. Am J Physiol 273: R755–R761

12. Daun JM, McCarthy DO (1993) The role of cholecystokinin in interleukin-1 induced anorexia. Physiol Behav 54: 237–241

13. Dryden S, Wang Q, Frankish HM et al. (1996) Differential effects of the 5-HT1B/2C receptor agonist mCPP and the 5-HT1A agonist flesinoxan on hypothalamic neuropeptide Y in the rat: evidence that NPY may mediate serotonin's effect on food intake. Peptides 17: 943–949

14. Elmstahl S, Persson M, Andren M et al. (1997) Malnutrition in geriatric patients: a neglected problem? J of Advanced Nursing 26: 851–855

15. Espat NJ, Auffenberg T, Rosenberg JJ et al. (1996) Ciliary neurotrophic factor is catabolic and shares with IL-6 the capacity to induce an acute phase response. Am J Physiol 271: R185–R190

16. Fagiolo U, Cosarizza A, Santacaterina S et al. (1992) Increased cytokine production by peripheral blood mononuclear cells from healthy elderly people. Ann NY Acad Sci 663: 490–493

17. Fantuzzi G, Benigni F, Sironi M et al. (1995) Ciliary neurotrophic factor (CNTF) induces serum amyloid A, hypoglyceaia and anorexia, and potentiates IL-1 induced corticosterone and IL-6 production in mice. Cytokine 7: 150–156

18. Feingold KR, Soued M, Adi S et al. (1991) Effect of interleukin-1 on lipid metabolism in the rate. Similarities to and differences from tumor necrosis factor. Arteriosclerosis & Thrombosis 11: 495–500

19. Ferraris RP, Vinnakota RR (1993) Regulation of intestinal nutrient transport is impaired in old mice. J Nutr 123: 502–511

20. Figlewikz DP, Stein LJ, Woods SC et al. (1985) Acute and chronic gastrin releasing peptide decreases food intake in baboons. Am J Physiol 248: R578–R583

21. Finck BN, Johnson RW (1997) Anorexia, weight loss and increased plasma interleukin-6 caused by chronic intracerebroventricular infusion of interleukin-1 beta in the rate. Brain Res 761: 333–337

22. Flores EA, Bristian BR, Pomposelli JJ et al. (1989) Infusion of tumor necrosis factor/ cachectin promotes muscle catabolism in the rat. A synergistic effect with interleukin 1. J Clin Invest 83: 1614–1622

23. Fried SK, Zechner R (1989) Cachectin/tumor necrosis factor decreases human adipose tissue lipoprotein lipase mRNA levels, synthesis, and activity. J Lipid Res 30: 1917–1923

24. Gershenwald JE, Fong YM, Fahey TJ et al. (1990) Interleukin 1 receptor blockage attenuates the host inflammatory response. Proc Natl Acad Sci USA 87: 4966–4970

25. Gosnell BA, Levine AS, Morley JE (1983) The effects of aging on opioid modulation of feeding in rats. Life Sci 32: 2793–2799

26. Greenberg RE, Holt PR (1986) Influence of aging upon pancreatic digestive enzymes. Digestive Diseases and Sciences 31: 970–977

27. Grunfield C, Zhao C, Fuller J et al. (1996) Endotoxin and cytokines induce expression of cytokines, the ob gene product, in hamsters. J Clin Invest 97: 2152–2157

28. Granowitz EV (1997) Transforming growth factor-beta enhances and pro-inflammatory cytokines inhibit OB gene expression in 3T3-L1 adipocytes. Biochemical and Biophysical Research Communications 240: 382–385

29. Gutzwiller JP, Drewe J, Hildebrand P et al. (1994) Effect of intravenous gastrin-releasing peptide on food intake in humans. Gastroenterology 106: 1168–1173

30. Hasselgren PO, Fisher JE (1998) Sepsis: Stimulation of protein-dependent breakdown resulting in protein loss in skeletal muscle. World J Surg 22: 203–208

31. Hill AG, Jacobson L, Gonzalez J et al. (1996) Chronic central nervous system exposure to interleukin-1 beta causes catabolism in rats. Am J Physiol 271: R1142–R1148

32. Ho LT, Chern YF, Lin MT (1989) The hypothalamic somatostatinergic pathways mediate feeding behavior in rats. Experientia 45: 161–162

33. Hotta M, Shibasaki T, Yamauchi N et al. (1991) The effects of chronic central administration of corticotrophin-releasing factor on food intake, body weight and hypothalamic-pituitary-adrenocortical hormones. Life Sci 48: 1483–1491

34. Janikk J, Curti BD, Considine RV et al. (1997) Interleukin 1 alpha increases serum leptin concentration in humans. J Clin Endocrinol Metab 82: 3084–3086

35. Kavaliers M, Teskey GC, Hirst M (1985) The effects of aging on day-night rhythms of kappa opiate-mediated feeding in the mouse. Psychopharmacology 87: 286–291

36. Kayali A, Young V, Goodman M (1987) Sensitivity of myofibrillar proteins to glucocorticoid-induced muscle proteolysis. Am J Physiol 252: E621

37. Lambert PD, Wilding JP, Al-Dokhayel AA et al. (1993) A role for neuropeptide-Y, dynorphin, and noradrenaline in the central control of food intake after deprivation. Endocrinology 133: 29–32

38. Leibowitz S, Weiss G, Suh J (1990) Medial hypothalamic nuclei mediate serotonin's inhibitory effect on feeding behaviour. Pharmac Biochem Behav 37: 735–742

39. Lieverse RJ, Janssen JB, Masclee AM et al. (1995) Effects of somatostatin on human satiety. Neuroendocrinology 61: 112–116

40. Lilic D, Cant AJ, Abinum M et al. (1997) Cytokine production differs in children and adults. Pediatr Res 42: 237–240

41. Ling PR, Schwartz JH, Bistrian BR (1997) Mechanisms of host wasting induced by administration of cytokines in rats. Am J Physiol 272: E333–E339

42. Llovera M, Garcia-Martinez C, Lopez-Soriano FJ et al. (1994) The effect of chronic tumor necrosis factor-alpha on urinary nitrogen excretion in the rat. Biochemistry & Molecular Biology International 3: 681–689

43. Lora-Vilchis MC, Chambert G, Rodriquez-Zendejas AM (1988) Ontogeny of alpha-and beta-adrenergic anorexia in rats. Am J Physiol 255: R908–913

44. Maltoni M, Fabbri L, Nanni O et al. (1997) Serum levels of tumor necrosis factor alpha and other cytokines do not correlate with weight loss and anorexia in cancer patients. Support Care Cancer 5: 130–135

45. Martin D, Merkel E, Tucker KK et al. (1996) Cachectic effect of ciliary neurotrophic factor on innervated skeletal muscle. Am J Physiol 271: R1422–R1428

46. Masclee AA, Geusken LM, Driessen WM et al. (1988) Effect of aging on plasma chole-cystokinin secretion and gallbladder emptying. Age 11: 136–140
47. Mizuno T, Bergen A, Kleopoulus S et al. (1996) Effects of nutritional status and aging on leptin gene expression in mice: Importance of glucose. Horm Metab Res 28: 679–684
48. Mooradian AD, Reed RL, Osterweil D et al. (1990) Lack of an association between the presence of tumor necrosis factor or interleukin-1 alpha in the blood and weight loss among elderly patients. J Am Geriatr Soc 38: 397–401
49. Morin CJ, Pagliassotti MJ, Windmiller D et al. (1997) Adipose-tissue derived tumor necrosis factor-alpha activity is elevated in older rats. J Gerontol 52: 190–195
50. Morley JE, Flood JF (1991) Amylin decreases food intake in mice. Peptides 12: 865–869
51. Morley JE, Flood JF (1992) Competitive antagonism of nitric oxide synthetase causes weight loss in mice. Life Sci 51: 1285–1289
52. Morley JE, Flood JF, Farr SA et al. (1995) Effects of amylin on appetite regulation and memory. Can J Physiol Pharmacol 73: 1042–1046
53. Morley JE, Flood JF, Silver AJ (1990) Opioid peptides and aging. Ann NY Acad Sci 579: 123–132
54. Morley JE, Kumar VB, Mattammal MB et al. (1996) Inhibition of feeding by a nitric oxide synthase inhibitor: Effects of aging. Eur J Pharmacol 311: 15–19
55. Morley JE, Perry HM, Kaiser FE et al. (1993) Longitudinal changes in testosterone, luteinizing hormone, and follicle stimulating hormone in healthy older males. J Am Geriatr Soc 41: 149–152
56. Morley JE, Suarez MD, Mattammal MB et al. (1997) Amylin and food intake in mice: effects on motivation eat and mechanism of action. Pharmacol Biochem Behav 56: 123–129
57. Oldenburg HS, Rogy MA, Lazarus DD et al. (1993) Cachexia and the acute-phase protein response in inflammation are related by interleukin-6. Eur J Immunol 23: 1889–1894
58. Plata-Salaman CR, Vaselli JR, Sonti G (1997) Differential responsiveness of obese (fa/fa) and lean (Fa/Fa) rats to cytokine-induced anorexia. Obes Res 5: 36–42
59. Poston GJ, Singh F, Draviam EJ et al. (1988) Development and age-related changes in pancreatic cholecystokinin receptors and duodenal cholecystokinin in guinea pigs. Mech Ageing Dev 46: 59–66
60. Rodriguez-Zendejas AM, Chambert G, Lora-Vilchis MC et al. (1986) Ontogeny of epinephrine-induced in rats. Am J Physiol 250: R303–R317
61. Roubenoff R, Roubenoff RA, Cannon JG et al. (1994) Rheumatoid cachexia: Cytokine-driven hypermetabolism accompanying reduced body cell mass in chronic inflammation. J Clin Invest 93: 2379–2386
62. Sakurai T, Amemiya A, Ishii M et al. (1998) Orexins and orexin receptors: A family of hypothalamic neuropeptides and G protein-coupled receptors that regulate feeding behavior. Cell 92: 573–585
63. Sarraf P, Frederich RC, Turner EM, et al. (1997) Multiple cytokines raise mouse leptin levels: Potential role in inflammatory anorexia. J Exp Med 185: 171–175
64. Schneider BS, Monahan JW, Hirsch J (1979) Brain cholecystokinin and nutritional status in rats and mice. Clin Invest 64: 1348–1356
65. Schwartz MW, Seeley RJ, Campfield LA et al. (1996) Identification of targets of leptin action in rat hypothalamus. J Clin Invest 98: 1101–1106
66. Silver AJ, Flood JF, Morley JE (1988) Effect of gastrointestinal peptides on ingestion in old and young mice. Peptides 9: 221–225
67. Siren AL, Liu Y, Feuerstein G et al. (1993) Increased release of tumor necrosis factor-alpha into the cerebrospinal fluid and peripheral circulation of aged rats. Stroke 24: 880–886
68. Sonti G, Ilyin SE, Plata-Salaman CR (1996) Anorexia induced by cytokine interactions at pathophysiological concentrations. Am J Physiol 270: R1394–R1402
69. Tessitore L, Costelli P, Baccino FM (1993) Humoral mediation for cachexia in tumour-bearing rats. Br J Cancer 67: 15–23
70. Uehara A. Sekiya C, Takasugi Y et al. (1989) Anorexia induced by interleukin 1: involvement of corticotrophin-releasing factor. Am J Physiol 257: R613–R617

71. Voigt JP, Huston JP, Voits M et al. (1996) Effects of cholecystokinin octapeptide (CCK-8) on food intake in adult and aged rats under different feeding conditions. Peptides 17: 1313–1315
72. Warren EJ, Finck BN, Arkins S et al. (1997) Coincidental changes in behavior and plasma cortisol in unrestrained pigs after intracerebroventricular injection of tumor necrosis factor-alpha. Endocrinology 138: 2365–2371
73. Xu B, Dube MG, Kalra PS et al. (1998) Anorectic effects of the cytokine, ciliary neurotrophic factor, are mediate by hypothalamic neuropeptide Y: Comparison with leptin. Endocrinology 139: 466–473
74. Yang ZJ, Koseki M. Meguid MM et al. (1994) Synergistic effect of rhTNF-alpha and rhIL-alpha in inducing anorexia in rats. Am J Physiol 267: R1056–R1064

Author's address:

John E. Morley, M.B., B.Ch.
Dammert Professor of Gerontology
Saint Louis University Health Sciences Center
Division of Geriatric Medicine
1402 S. Grand Boulevard, Room M238
St. Louis, MO 63104, USA

Aging and water metabolism in health and illness

M. Miller

Departments of Medicine, Levindale Hebrew Geriatric Center and Hospital, Sinai Hospital of Baltimore and the Johns Hopkins University School of Medicine, Baltimore, MD, USA

Summary

Normal aging is associated with changes in body composition, thirst perception, renal function, and the hormonal regulatory systems involved in the maintenance of water and sodium balance. The presence of many diseases and drugs common in the elderly can interact with the impaired homeostatic systems to result in clinically significant disturbances of water and sodium with accompanying symptoms, morbidity, and mortality. These disorders, which include dehydration, hypernatremia, hyponatremia, urinary frequency, and urinary incontinence can either be prevented or promptly recognized and appropriately treated by understanding the physiological changes and clinical circumstances which put the elderly person at increased risk for deranged water and sodium balance.

Introduction

Nutrition is commonly thought of in terms of food intake with such components as calories, carbohydrates, proteins, fats, vitamins, and minerals. Less often is the fluid component of dietary intake considered even though the maintenance of health and body function requires that the composition of fluid and electrolyte compartments be maintained within a narrow range. The ability to regulate water and electrolyte balance involves the interplay of a number of homeostatic systems, many of which can be compromised by the normal aging process itself or by diseases or drugs commonly present in the elderly (27). Thus, when the older person is challanged by disease, drugs or impaired ability to gain access to or to control intake of fluid, the result may be water retention or loss and hyponatremia or hypernatremia with symptomatic consequences.

Normal aging effects on fluid regulatory systems (Table 1)

Body composition

Normal aging is accompanied by a decrease in lean body mass, an increase in fat, and a decrease in total body water from approximately 60 % of body weight in

Table 1. Aging effects on sodium and water regulatory systems

Body composition	Decreased total body water Decreased intracellular fluid compartment	
Fluid intake	Decreased thirst perception	
Hormonal systems	Vasopressin	Normal or increased basal secretion Increased response to osmotic stimulation Decreased nocturnal secretion
	Atrial natriuretic hormone	Increased basal secretion Increased response to stimulation
	Decreased plasma renin activity Decreased aldosterone production	
Renal function	Decreased kidney mass Decline in renal blood flow Decline in glomerular filtration rate Impaired distal renal tubular diluting capacity Impaired renal concentrating capacity Impaired sodium conservation Impaired renal response to vasopressin	

young men and 52 % in young women to 54 % and 46 %, respectively, in individuals over the age of 65 years. The decrease in total body water takes place primarily in the intracellular fluid compartment. This change in body composition has the potential to contribute to derangements in fluid balance including dehydration and/or hypernatremia when the older person is challanged by fluid loss or decreased fluid intake and fluid overload and hyponatremia when exposed to excessive oral or parenteral fluid intake.

Fluid requirements

Under normal conditions, the requirement for daily fluid intake is approximately 30 ml/kg body weight. The presence of increased environmental temperature, fever, decreased fluid intake or increased gastrointestinal, urinary or respiratory fluid loss places the elderly person at risk for dehydration with consequences which can be life threatening if suitable increase in fluid intake is not accomplished. Similarly, the elderly person who is exposed to increased amounts of fluid either orally or by parenteral routes must be closely monitored to avoid development of symptomatic levels of hyponatremia.

Thirst perception

The ability to ingest sufficient fluid to meet body needs requires that thirst perception be present and that the individual is physically capable of obtaining and consuming a suitable source of fluid. The control of thirst resides in the central nervous system and is regulated by both extracellular fluid volume and tonicity with plasma osmolality being the most important factor in the day to day perception of thirst. In young, healthy persons, thirst is usually stimulated when the plasma osmolality rises to values greater than 292 mOsm/kg (37) . Healthy older persons over the age of 65 years have shown evidence for an age-associated impairment in thirst sensation so that when they are subjected to water deprivation sufficient to raise plasma osmolality to greater than 296 mOsm/kg, they exhibit much less thirst and water consumption than young persons who have been similarly water deprived (34). In addition to this effect of normal aging, patients with cerebrovascular accidents also may have a profound impairment in thirst perception even in the presence of volume depletion and hyperosmolality (31).

Hormonal regulation of water and sodium

Among the major factors in the ability of the body to closely regulate fluid balance are the hypothalamic hormone arginine vasopressin or antidiuretic hormone (AVP, ADH) which acts on the kidney to control water excretion, atrial natriuretic hormone (ANH) which is released from the myocardium and acts on the kidney to cause natriuresis, and the renin-angiotensin-aldosterone system which acts on the kidney to conserve sodium. All of these hormonal systems are affected by the normal aging process (26).

Arginine vasopressin

There is much evidence based on histologic examination of the hypothalamus which indicates that activity of the AVP system not only does not decline during normal aging, but actually may increase with age (16, 20). Clinically, basal blood levels of AVP do not appear to be affected by aging (8, 12) although there may be an age-related loss of the normal nocturnal rise in AVP secretion (3). In response to the stimulus of hyperosmolality, older persons have been found to exhibit a greater increase in blood AVP than occurs in younger persons (19, 34). Similarly, pharmacologic stimulation of AVP release by metoclopramide or by physostigmine results in a greater response in older persons (7, 36). These studies suggest that the older person may be at increased risk for development of water retention and hyponatremia such as is seen in the syndrome of inappropriate secretion of antidiuretic hormone (SIADH) when they are challanged by stimuli capable of causing the release of AVP.

Atrial natriuretic hormone

ANH is synthesized and stored in the atria of the heart where it is released into the circulation in response to increase in intracardiac pressure and acts on the kidney to produce a natriuresis and accompanying diuresis (14). There is an age-related increase in basal levels of ANH in the blood and the elderly exhibit an exaggerated response of ANH to stimuli which increase intracardiac pressure such as acute intravascular volume expansion and exercise-induced tachycardia (32). Not only is there an increased release of ANH in the elderly, but there is also evidence that the renal natriuretic response to ANH may be greater in the older person than in the young (18).

In addition to its direct natriuretic action, ANH also suppresses renal renin secretion, plasma renin activity, plasma angiotensin II generation, and aldosterone secretion from the adrenal gland (10). Thus, ANH may be an important mediator of age-associated renal sodium loss, both directly through its renal natriuretic action and indirectly through suppression of aldosterone secretion.

Renin-angiotensin-aldosterone

Study of healthy older persons has demonstrated that the aging process is associated with a decrease in the activity of the renin-angiotensin-aldosterone system both under basal conditions and after stimulation by upright posture and sodium depletion (6, 44). The mechanisms responsible include impaired conversion of inactive to active renin and the inhibitory effects of increased amounts of ANH on renin secretion. The consequence of decreased aldosterone secretion is an impairment in renal sodium conserving ability and an increase in the risk for the development of hyperkalemia (35).

Renal water and sodium regulation

Renal structural and functional changes

Renal mass declines progressively with age and is accompanied by a decrease in the number of glomeruli, a decrease in effective filtering surface, an increase in mesangial cells, a decrease in number of epithelial cells, and thickening of the glomerular basement membrane (21). Renal blood flow declines by approximately 10 % per decade after young adulthood so that by age 90 years there is a reduction to about 50 % of the value found at age 30 years (11). In association with these changes, glomerular filtration rate begins to decline after age 40 years at an annual rate of 0.8 ml/min per 1.73 M^2 (39). There is much individual variability so that not all aging persons undergo a decline in glomerular filtration rate.

Water regulation

The decline in glomerular filtration rate is associated with an alteration in renal diluting capacity. In response to acute water loading, there is an age-related impairment in ability to reduce urine osmolality (23). These changes can lead to increased reabsorption of fluid with the consquent risk of water overload and dilutional hyponatremia.

Aging is also associated with an impairment in renal concentrating capacity. In response to water deprivation, older persons show a decrease in the maximum attainable urine osmolality and in the ability to decrease urine flow (39). The impaired concentration is at least partially due to decreased renal responsiveness to AVP (25).

Sodium regulation

The age-related decrease in renal blood flow and glomerular filtration rate can lead to enhanced renal conservation of sodium with an accompanying water retention. This effect on sodium handling is further enhanced in the presence of diseases common in the elderly such as congestive heart failure, cirrhosis or renal insufficiency. Drugs such as nonsteroidal antiinflamatory agents can promote sodium retention and increase the risk for congestive heart failure (17). The ability of the aging kidney to efficiently conserve sodium can also be impaired. In response to restricted dietary sodium intake, older persons take a much greater time to decrease urinary sodium excretion than do young individuals (13).

Disorders of fluid regulation

As a consequence of the aging effects on water and sodium homeostatic systems, the elderly person is at increased risk of developing clinically significant disturbances of water and sodium balance in response to many common stresses, diseases or drugs.

Table 2. Risk factors for hypernatremia in the elderly

Increased water loss	Renal
	Age-associated impaired concentrating capacity
	Resistance to vasopressin action Age-associated
	Acquired (drugs, hypokalemia, hypercalcemia)
	Osmotic diuresis (glycosuria, diuretic-induced natriuresis)
	Renal tubular disease
	Gastrointestinal tract
	Vomiting
	Diarrhea
	Skin (sweating)
	Lung (tachypnea)
Decreased water intake	Impaired thirst perception
	Impaired cognition (delerium, dementia)
	Impaired access to fluids

Hypernatremia

Approximately 1 % of hospitalized patients over the age of 60 years have been found to have hypernatremia (42). Elderly persons residing in nursing homes are at even higher risk with as many as 34 % developing dehyration and hypernatremia when they acquire an acute illness (22). Most commonly, hypernatremia is the result of loss of body water in excess of sodium loss in association with inadequate fluid intake (Table 2). Frequent causes are febrile illness with confusion and decreased food and fluid intake along with increased insensible fluid loss, tachypnea with increased water loss from the lungs, gastrointestinal fluid loss from vomiting or diarrhea, and osmotically-induced urine excretion from use of diuretics or from poorly controlled diabetes mellitus. Patients with Alzheimer's disease have decreased thirst perception and are at high risk for dehydration (1). The clinical consequences of dehydration and hypernatremia in the elderly are significant and include alterations in level of consciousness, cardiovascular collapse, renal failure, and death, especially when serum sodium concentration is greater than 148 mEq/L (33, 42).

Hyponatremia

Hyponatremia occurs when there is an alteration in the relationship between the amount of sodium and water in the extracellular body fluid compartment as a result of either a decrease in extracellualar sodium content (sodium depletion) or

Table 3. Risk factors for hyponatremia in the elderly

Physiologic changes of normal aging	Water Retention	Decreased renal blood flow and glomerular filtration rate Decreased distal renal tubular diluting capacity Increased renal passive reabsorption of water Increased vasopressin secretion
	Sodium Loss	Altered renal tubular function Increased Atrial Natriuretic Hormone Secretion Decreased renin-angiotensin-aldosterone secretion
Increased water intake	Oral Fluids Intravenous Hypotonic Fluids	
Decreased sodium intake	Low Sodium Diet Tube Feeding	
Increased sodium loss	Renal Disease Gastrointestinal Tract: Vomiting, Diarrhea, Gastric suctioning	
Idiopathic SIADH* of the elderly	Age > 80 Years Race Other Than Black	

*SIADH = Syndrome of Inappropriate Antidiuretic Hormone Secretion

Table 4. Diseases associated with hyponatremia in the elderly

Central nervous system disorders	Vascular Diseases Trauma (Subdural Hematoma, Intracranial Hemorrhage) Tumor Infectious Disease
Malignancy with ectopic AVP production	Pulmonary (Small Cell Carcinoma) Pancreatic Carcinoma Thymoma Lymphosarcoma, Reticulum Cell Sarcoma, Hodgkin's Disease
Pulmonary disease	Pneumonia Tuberculosis Lung Abscess Bronchiectasis
Endocrine disease	Hypothyroidism Diabetes Mellitus with Hyperglycemia Adrenal Insufficiency

an increase in extracellular water (dilutional hyponatremia). The physiologic changes that take place in water regulation during aging may be clinically expressed in the very old as hyponatremia which has the characteristics of the syndrome of inappropriate antidiuretic hormone secretion (SIADH) (28). Hyponatremia is a common finding in the elderly, with prevalence ranging from 7 % in community residing older persons to more than 20 % of residents in long-term care institutions (29). A number of factors have been identified which, in association with normal aging effects on water and sodium regulation, increase the risk for hyponatremia (Table 3).

Altered water and sodium intake

The administration of hypotonic fluid either as an increase in oral water intake or as intravenous infusion of 0.45 % saline solution or 5 % glucose in water has been found to be a major factor in the development or worsening of hyponatremia in 78 % of nursing home residents with the disorder (29). Low sodium intake can lead to sodium depletion with consequent hyponatremia, especially in patients whose nutritional support is primarily or entirely provided by tube feeding since the sodium content is low in many of the tube feeding preparations (29, 40).

Diseases and hyponatremia

Disease states such as congestive heart failure, cirrhosis, and primary renal failure are often accompanied by a decrease in effective intravascular volume with decreased renal blood flow and glomerular filtration rate and can result in retention

Table 5. Drug-induced changes in sodium and water regulation

Sodium retention	Non-steroidal anti-inflamatory agents
Sodium loss	Thiazide and loop diuretics
Impaired diluting capacity	Thiazide diuretics
Impaired concentrating capacity	Lithium Demeclocycline Potassium-losing diuretics

Syndrome of inappropriate antidiuretic hormone secretion	Central Nervous System Agents
	  Tricyclic antidepressants
	  Selective serotonin reuptake inhibitor
	    antidepressants
	  Phenothiazine antipsychotics
	  Carbamazepine anticonvulsant
	Angiotensin Converting Enzyme (ACE) Inhibitors
	Antineoplastic drugs
	  Vincristine
	  Vinblastine
	Cyclophosphamide
	Chlorpropamide
	Clofibrate
	Narcotics

of water in excess of sodium with consequent hyponatremia (Table 4). Especially common in the elderly are diseases in which the cause of hyponatremia is SIADH. Almost all central nervous system disorders can lead to hypothalamic dysfunction with increased AVP secretion and consequent risk for water retention and hyponatremia (5). These disorders include vascular injury (thrombosis, embolism hemorrhage), trauma with subdural hematoma, vasculitis, tumor, and infection. Malignancy can cause SIADH by release into the circulation of AVP synthesized in cancer tissue. The most common such malignancy is small cell carcinoma of the lung in which as many as 68 % of patients have been found to have evidence of impaired water excretion (9). Other cancers which can cause SIADH include pancreatic carcinoma, thymoma, pharyngeal carcinoma, lymphosarcoma, and Hodgkins disease. Inflamatory lung disease such as pneumonia, bronchiectasis, lung abscess, and tuberculosis can also cause SIADH, possibly as a result of AVP production and release by the diseased pulmonary tissue.

Hypothyroidism and adrenal insufficiency may be accompanied by hyponatremia with features of SIADH. Non-SIADH mechanisms such as altered renal tubular water reabsorption and renal sodium loss can also contribute to hyponatremia in these conditions. Poorly controlled diabetes mellitus with marked hyperglycemia can cause redistribution of body water into the intravascular space with resultant dilutional decrease of serum sodium of approximately 1.6 mEq/L for each 100 mg/100 ml increase in blood sugar over normal.

Drugs and hyponatremia

Numerous drugs (Table 5) taken by elderly persons can cause hyponatremia by enhancing the release of AVP from the neurohypophyseal system or by increasing renal sodium loss. Central nervous system acting drugs are especially likely to cause SIADH and include tricyclic and serotonin reuptake inhibitor antidepressants, antipsychotics, and the anticonvulsant carbamazepine (24, 30).

Angiotensin-converting enzyme (ACE) inhibitors have been associated with the development of SIADH-type hyponatremia in elderly patients. The level of hyponatremia can be clinically significant with serum sodium concentration as low as 101 mEq/L and with symptoms of confusion, seizures, and coma (43). Stopping the ACE inhibitor results in rapid resolution of the hyponatremia.

Both thiazide and loop diuretics can produce significant hyponatremia. When diuretic-induced sodium and water loss is replaced by hypotonic fluids, a combined depletional and dilutional hyponatremia will be the result. Thiazide-induced hyponatremia is often accompanied by loss of total body potassium and hypokalemia which can lead to activation of hypothalamic pathways involved in AVP discharge and the development of SIADH. This circumstance occurs almost entirely in the elderly and can be corrected by appropriate potassium replacement (15).

Other drugs associated with SIADH in the elderly include the sulfonylurea chlorpropamide, and the antineoplastic agents vincristine, vinblastine, and cyclophosphamide. Narcotics can be responsible for hyponatremia in the elderly postoperative patient.

Nocturia and urinary incontinence

In many older persons there is loss of the nocturnal rise in AVP which normally occurs in the young (3). As a result, there is a reversal of day/night urine production so that nighttime urine flow rate exceeds the daytime flow rate with a diabetes insipidus-like nocturnal poluria (2). When coupled with the diminished bladder capacity and detrussor hyper-reflexia so common in older persons, the result is nocturnal urinary frequency. In the presence of impaired mobility or cognition, nocturnal frequency can be converted to urinary incontinence. It is possible that the AVP analog DDAVP may be helpful in the treatment of both nocturnal frequency and urinary incontinence (4, 41).

Conclusion

The age-associated changes in water and sodium regulatory systems which occur as part of normal aging put the elderly person at increased risk for the development of disorders of water and sodium balance. The further challange of diseases, disabilities, and drugs common in the elderly can result in clinically significant symptoms with accompanying morbidity and mortality. Attention to the nutritional water and sodium needs of the older person can either prevent disturbances of water balance or allow prompt recognition and initiation of appropriate interventions.

References

1. Albert SG, Nakra BRS, Grossberg GT et al. (1994) Drinking behavior and vasopressin responses to hyperosmolality in Alzheimer's disease. Int Psychogeriatrics 6: 78–86
2. Asplund R (1995) The nocturnal polyuria syndrome (NPS). Gen Pharmac 26: 1203–1209
3. Asplund R, Aberg H (1991) Diurnal variation in the levels of antidiuretic hormone in the elderly. J Intern Med 299: 131–134
4. Asplund R, Aberg H (1993) Desmopressin in elderly subjects with increased nocturnal diuresis. A two-month treatment study. Scand J Urol Nephrol 27: 77–82
5. Bartter FC, Schwartz WB (1967) The syndrome of inappropriate secretion of antidiuretic hormone. Am J Med 42: 790–806
6. Bauer JH (1993) Age-related changes in the renin-aldosterone system. Physiological effects and clinical implications. Drugs Ageing 3: 238–245
7. Bevilacqua M, Norbiato G, Chebat E et al. (1987) Osmotic and nonosmotic control of vaso- pressin release in the elderly: effect of metoclopramide. J Clin Endocrinol Metab 54: 1243–1247
8. Chiodera P, Capretti L, Marches M (1991) Abnormal arginine vasopressin response to cigarette smoking and metoclopramide (but not to insulin-induced hypoglycemia) in elderly subjects. J Gerontol 46: M6–M10
9. Comis RL, Miller M, Ginsberg SJ (1980) Abnormalities in water homeostasis in small cell anaplastic lung cancer. Cancer 45: 2414–2421
10. Cuneo RC, Espiner EA, Nicholls MG et al. (1987) Effect of physiological levels of atrial natriuretic peptide on hormone secretion: inhibition of angiotensin-induced aldosterone secretion and renin release in normal man. J Clin Endocrinol Metab 65: 765–772
11. Davies DF, Shock NW (1950) Age changes in glomerular filtration, effective renal plasma flow and tubular excretory capacity in adult males. J Clin Invest 29: 496–506
12. Duggan J, Kilfeather S, Lightman SL et al. (1993) The association of age with plasma arginine vasopressin and plasma osmolality. Age Ageing 22: 332–336
13. Epstein M, Hollenberg NK (1976) Age as a determinant of renal sodium conservation in normal man. J Lab Clin Med 87: 411–417
14. Espiner EA, Richards AM, Yandle TG, Nicholls MG (1995) Natriuretic hormones. Endo- crinology Metab Clinics N Am 24: 481–509
15. Fichman MP, Vorherr H, Kleeman CR et al. (1971) Diuretic-induced hyponatremia. Ann Intern Med 75: 853–863
16. Fliers E, Swaab DF, Pool Ch W et al. (1985) The vasopressin and oxytocin neurons in the human supraoptic and paraventricular nucleus: change with aging and in senile dementia. Brain Res 342: 45–53
17. Heerdink ER, Leufkens HG, Herings RMC, Ottervanger JP, Stricker BHC, Bakker A (1998) NSAIDs associated with increased risk of congestive heart failure in elderly patients taking diuretics. Arch Intern Med 158: 1108–1112
18. Heim JM, Gottmann JW, Strom TM, Gerzer R (1989) Effects of a bolus dose of atrial natriuretic factor in young and elderly volunteers. Eur J Clin Invest 19: 265–271
19. Helderman JH, Vestal RE, Rowe JW et al. (1978) The response of arginine vasopressin to intra- venous ethanol and hypertonic saline in man. The impact of aging. J gerontol 33: 39–47
20. Hoogendijk JE, Fliers E, Swaab DF et al. (1985) Activation of vasopressin neurons in the human supraoptic and paraventricular nucleus in senescence and senile dementia. J Neurol Sci 69: 291–299
21. Kappel B, Olsen S (1980) Cortical interstitial tissue and sclerosed glomeruli in the normal human kidney, related to age and sex. Virchows Arch (A) 387: 271–277
22. Lavizo-Mourey R, Johnson J, Stolley P (1988) Risk factors for dehydration among elderly nursing home residents. J Am Geriatr Soc 36: 213–218
23. Lindeman RD, Lee DT, Yiengst MJ, Shock NW (1966) Influence of age, renal disease, hyper- tension, diuretics and calcium on the antidiuretic responses to suboptimal infusions of vasopressin. J Lab Clin Med 68: 202–223

24. Liu BA, Mittmann N, Knowles SR, Shear NH (1996) Hyponatremia and the syndrome of inappropriate secretion of antidiuretic hormone associated with the use of selective serotonin reuptake inhibitors: a review of spontaneous reports. Canadian Med Assoc J 155: 519–527

25. Miller JH, Shock NW (1953) Age differences in the renal tubular response to antidiuretic hormone. J Gerontol 8: 446–450

26. Miller M (1995) Hormonal aspects of fluid and sodium balance in the elderly. Endocrinology Metab Clinics N Am 24: 233–253

27. Miller M, Gold GC, Friedlander DA (1991) Physiological changes of aging affecting salt and water balance. Rev Clin Gerontology 1: 215–230

28. Miller M, Hecker MS, Friedlander DA, Carter JM (1996) Apparent idiopathic hyponatremia in an ambulatory geriatric population. J Am Geriatr Soc 44: 404–408

29. Miller M, Morley JE, Rubenstein LZ (1995) Hyponatremia in a nursing home population. J Am Geriatr Soc 43: 1410–1413

30. Miller M, Moses AM (1976) Drug-induced states of impaired water excretion. Kidney Int 10: 96–103

31. Miller PD, Krebs RA, Neal BJ, McIntyre DO (1982) Hypodipsia in geriatric patients. Am J Med 73: 354–356

32. Ohashi M, Fujio N, Nawata H et al. (1987) High plasma concentrations of human atrial natriuretic polypepetide in aged men. J Clin Endocrinol Metab 64: 81–85

33. Palevsky PM, Bhagrath R, Greenberg A (1996) Hypernatremia in hospitalized patients. Ann Intern Med 124: 197–203

34. Phillips PA, Rolls BJ, Ledingham JGG et al. (1984) Reduced thirst after water deprivation in healthy elderly men. N Engl J Med 311: 753–759

35. Ponce SP, Jennings AS, Madias, NE et al. (1985) Drug-induced hyperkalemia. Medicine 64: 357–370

36. Raskind MA, Peskind ER, Veith RC et al. (1989) Neuroendocrine responses to physostigmine in Alzheimer's disease. Arch Gen Psychiatry 46: 535–540

37. Robertson GL (1983) Thirst and vasopressin function in normal and disordered states of water balance. J Lab Clin Med 101: 351–371

38. Rowe JW, Andres RA, Tobin JD et al. (1976) The effect of age on creatinine clearance in man: a cross-sectional and longitudinal study. J Gerontol 311: 155–163

39. Rowe JW, Shock NW, DeFronzo RA (1976) The influence of age on the renal response to water deprivation in man. Nephron 17: 270–278

40. Rudman D, Racette D, Rudman IW et al. (1986) Hyponatremia in tube-fed elderly men. J Chronic Dis 39: 73–80

41. Seiler WO, Stahelin HB, Hefti U (1992) Desmopressin reduces night urine volume in geriatric patients: implications for treatment of the nocturnal incontinence. Clin Invest 70: 619

42. Snyder NA, Feigel DW, Arieff AI (1987) Hypernatremia in elderly patients. A heterogeneous, morbid, and iatrogenic entity. Ann Intern Med 107: 309–319

43. Subramanian D, Ayus JC (1992) Case report: severe symptomatic hyponatremia associated with lisinopril therapy. Am J Med Sci 303: 177–179

44. Weidmann P, DeMyttenaere-Bursztein S, Maxwell MH et al. (1975) Effect of aging on plasma renin and aldosterone in normal man. Kidney Int 8: 325–333

Author's address:

Myron Miller, M.D.
Sinai Hospital of Baltimore
2401 West Belvedere Avenue
Baltimore, MD 21215-5271, USA
E-mail: myrmiller@pol.net

Malnutrition and mental functions*

H. B. Stähelin

Geriatrische Universitätsklinik, Kantonsspital, Basel, Switzerland

Summary

Prolonged suboptimal intake of micronutrients leads via a series of mechanisms to impairment of cognitive performance. Supplementation can correct these deficits. Malnutrition impairs cognitive performance only when micronutrient levels fall below certain critical thresholds. Malnutrition in the elderly is commonly the result of preexisting mental impairment due to chronic diseases. These also lead to accelerated neuronal destruction via a stress response of the hypothalamic-pituitary-adrenal axis. Subtle dietary deficits can lead over many years to quantifiable impairment of cognitive performance. Severe dietary deficiency leading to major cognitive impairment is nevertheless rare.

Introduction

As compared with other bodily functions, mental functions are relatively little affected by age-related physiological changes. Memory, emotionality, and mental performance are retained until a very advanced age in healthy individuals. Only the rapidity of thought processes is subject to a marked aging effect. Preservation of mental functions is one of the principal preconditions for retention of autonomy and independence in the elderly. Despite the existence of great reserves and physiological safety mechanisms, preservation of mental functions in the elderly is dependent not just on energy and oxygen intake, but also, both directly and indirectly, on an adequate intake of micronutrients.

Symptoms such as forgetfulness and irritability, and also definite neurological signs, can occur in various vitamin deficiency states. If not identified, they can lead to irreversible damage (3). Above-average intake of vitamins and other micronutrients appears to delay the development of degenerative diseases (9, 12). By contrast, inadequate intake of these substances can significantly promote the development of chronic diseases and, thus, impair the health of the elderly

---

* This contribution was translated from German to English by David Playfair, 30 Cheverton Road, London N19 3AY, Great Britain, Email: DavidPlayfair@compuserve.com

population (1). Of particular importance in this respect is the impairment of mental functions that can result from many chronic degenerative brain diseases. Poor dietary habits in early and later adulthood can thus lead both directly and indirectly to impairment of mental function at a more advanced age.

Nutrient requirements are influenced by age, height, body composition, climate, sex, physical activity, diseases, and many other factors (13). With increasing age, consumption of food and, thus, also of energy and micronutrients falls, and the risk of malnutrition and specific dietary deficiencies rises. Elderly people find it increasingly difficult to maintain a balanced diet, and the likelihood of inadequate intake of essential micronutrients is further increased by great variability in the nutrient density of food.

At a conceptual level, dietary deficiencies might influence mental functions in any of three possible ways:

▶ by influencing the aging process at the cellular level and at the level of the organism;
▶ by promoting or preventing the development of chronic diseases;
▶ by direct action on cerebral function.

Aging of the brain, and thus the preservation of cognitive functions, is influenced by, among other things, the ability to deal with oxidative stress. Neurons, being postmitotic cells with a high energy turnover, are constantly exposed to oxidative processes (23). A causal role has been ascribed to oxidative stress in a number of age-related degenerative brain diseases including Alzheimerís disease and Parkinson's disease (6). The same is true of atherosclerosis (9), in which not only neurons, but also the major arteries that supply the brain, are affected. Vascular occlusions due to atherosclerotic plaques and thromboembolic events impair the blood supply to the brain and may, thus, become manifest as cognitive deficits. A number of studies have shown that a reduced intake of antioxidative micronutrients leads to an increased incidence of cerebrovascular events (8, 24).

In addition to antioxidative vitamins, other nutrients that may exert a protective effect include folic acid, vitamin B_{12}, and other bioactive secondary nutrients such as flavonoids, phyto-oestrogens, etc. (1). It should be emphasized that such substances have been found to influence the progression of chronic diseases not just in individuals with definite deficiencies of micronutrients – a group that accounts for only a very small proportion of European populations – but also to a significant extent in individuals with nutrient intakes in the lower part of the normal range (22).

An inadequate intake of micronutrients can, thus, hasten the development of neurodegenerative diseases. Certainly, there is a correlation between dietary intake and cognitive performance (11, 14, 21). Plasma vitamin C and carotene levels correlate with cognitive test scores and in particular with certain memory functions. Results similar to those obtained in the Basel study (21) were obtained also in the Rotterdam study (14) and in the SENECA study (11). Overall, lifelong administration of vitamins, and in particular antioxidative vitamins, appears to provide a degree of protection against neurodegenerative diseases and in this way leads to better retention of cognitive functions in the elderly (5, 10, 17). An intake that is low without actually being deficient can lead to significantly poorer mental function with increasing age. These effects must be clearly distinguished from the impairment of cognitive functions that occurs in individuals with a low vitamin B1 intake associated with chronic alcohol abuse (Wernicke's encephalopathy) and from that seen in clinical deficiency of vitamin B_{12}, vitamin B_6, or folic acid (3).

Inadequate vitamin intake in the elderly

Even under extreme circumstances, mental functions are very well preserved. Severe disturbance of mental functions, therefore, tends to occur only in individuals with definite nutritional deficiencies. Reference was made above to the indirect effects of nutritional deficiencies via chronic degenerative diseases. Only in the past few years has increasing interest been shown in the relationships between specific nutritional deficiencies and cognitive impairments in the elderly. Thus, relationships between neuropsychiatric disorders and B_{12} and folic acid metabolism have been described (4, 7), and a number of indicators clearly show the danger of inadequate intake of micronutrients (15, 18, 20). Overall, the concept of a threshold below which levels must fall before effects occur would appear to be valid in the case of acute functional disturbances, whereas in that of chronic disturbances the dose-effect principle would appear to be more valid. Thus, Wahlin et al. (25) observed better cognitive functions in individuals whose plasma vitamin B_{12} level was above 200 pmol/l than in those with lower levels. From this the authors concluded that "normal" plasma levels are adequate for cognitive function.

Disturbances of mental function and malnutrition due to metabolic changes

A number of studies have found a correlation between behavioral disturbances and low cholesterol levels. In one such study (19), low cholesterol levels were found to correlate with low Mini-Mental State Examination (MMSE) scores. This may be regarded as evidence that cognitive deficits correlate with evidence of malnutrition. Similarly, La Rue et al. (17) observed better cognitive performance in individuals with higher plasma levels and dietary intake of the B vitamins, folic acid, and vitamin C. Also significant is the finding that individuals who took vitamin supplements at their own initiative performed better in mental tests (2).

On the other hand, the complexity of the relationships between dietary deficiencies, stress, and cognition can be seen from the study by Kalmijn et al. (16). These authors found a statistically significant reduction in cognitive performance in individuals under stress. The relationships between mental functions and malnutrition are, thus, exceedingly complex, and mental impairments associated with malnutrition are not necessarily amenable to simple supplementation. In one study, elderly individuals with adequate cognitive functions were found to have a relatively low intake of fat and cholesterol and a relatively high intake of fruit, vegetables, carbohydrates, and the micronutrients referred to above (20).

In summary, prolonged suboptimal intake of micronutrients leads via a series of mechanisms to impairment of cognitive performance. Supplementation can correct these deficits. Malnutrition impairs cognitive performance only when micronutrient levels fall below certain critical thresholds. Malnutrition in the elderly is commonly the result of preexisting mental impairment due to chronic diseases. These also lead to accelerated neuronal destruction via a stress response of the hypothalamic-pituitary-adrenal axis. Subtle dietary deficits can lead over many years to quantifiable impairment of cognitive performance. Severe dietary deficiency leading to major cognitive impairment is nevertheless rare.

Literatur

1. The American Cancer Society 1996 Advisory Committee on Diet, Nutrition, and Cancer Prevention (1996) Guidelines on diet, nutrition, and cancer prevention: reducing the risk of cancer with healthy food choices and physical activity. Ca Cancer J Clin 46 (6): 325–41
2. Benton D, Griffiths R, Haller J (1997) Thiamine supplementation, mood and cognitive functioning. Psychopharmacology (Berlin) 129 (1): 66–71
3. Biesalski HK, Schrezenmeir J, Weber P, Weiss H (1997) Vitamine: Physiologie, Pathophysiologie, Therapie. Stuttgart: Georg Thieme
4. Bottiglieri T (1996) Folate, vitamin B_{12}, and neuropsychiatric disorders. Nutr Rev 54 (12): 382–90
5. Chome J, Paul T, Pudel V et al. (1986) Effects of suboptimal vitamin status on behavior. Bibl Nutr Dieta (Switzerland) 38: 94–103
6. de Rijk M, Breteler MM, den Breeijen J et al. (1997) Dietary antioxidants and Parkinson disease. The Rotterdam Study. Arch Neurol 54 (6): 762–5
7. Fava M, Borus JS, Alpert JE, Nierenberg AA, Rosenbaum JF, Bottiglieri T (1997) Folate, vitamin B_{12}, and homocysteine in major depressive disorder. Am J Psychiatry 154 (3): 426–8
8. Gale CR, Martyn CN, Cooper C (1996) Cognitive impairment and mortality in a cohort of elderly people. Br Med J 312 (7031): 608–11
9. Gey KF (1998) Vitamins E plus C and interacting conutrients required for optimal health. A critical and constructive review of epidemiology and supplementation data regarding cardiovascular disease and cancer. Biofactors 7 (1-2): 113–74
10. Goodwin JS, Goodwin JM, Garry PJ (1983) Association between nutritional status and cognitive functioning in a healthy elderly population. JAMA 249 (21): 2917–21
11. Haller J, Weggemans RM, Ferry M, Guigoz Y (1996) Mental health: minimental state examination and geriatric depression score of elderly Europeans in the SENECA study of 1993. Eur J Clin Nutr S112–6
12. Helzlsouer KJ, Block G, Blumberg J et al. (1994) Summary of the round table discussion on strategies for cancer prevention: diet, food, additives, supplements, and drugs. Cancer Res 54 (7 Suppl): 2044s–2051s
13. Heseker H (1997) Vitaminbedarf im Alter. In: Biesalski HK, Schrezenmeir J, Weber P, Weiss H (eds) Vitamine: Physiologie, Pathophysiologie, Therapie. Stuttgart: Georg Thieme
14. Jama JW, Launer LJ, Witteman JC et al. (1996) Dietary antioxidants and cognitive function in a population-based sample of older persons. The Rotterdam Study. Am J Epidemiol 144 (3): 275–80
15. Joosten E, A. vdB, Riezler R et al. (1993) Metabolic evidence that deficiencies of vitamin B_{12} (cobalamin), folate, and vitamin B_6 occur commonly in elderly people. Am J Clin Nutr 58 (4): 468–76
16. Kalmijn S, Feskens EJ, Launer LJ, Kromhout D (1997) Polyunsaturated fatty acids, antioxidants, and cognitive function in very old men. Am J Epidemiol 145 (1): 33–41

17. La Rue A, Koehler KM, Wayne SJ, Chiulli SJ, Haaland KY, Garry PJ (1997) Nutritional status and cognitive functioning in a normally aging sample: a 6-year reassessment [see comments]. Am J Clin Nutr 65 (1): 20–9

18. Lindenbaum J, Rosenberg IH, Wilson PW, Stabler SP, Allen RH (1994) Prevalence of cobalamin deficiency in the Framingham elderly population [see comments]. Am J Clin Nutr 60 (1): 2–11

19. Orengo CA, Kunik ME, Molinari VA, Teasdale TA, Workman RH, Yudofsky SC (1996) Association of serum cholesterol and triglyceride levels with agitation and cognitive function in a geropsychiatry unit. J Geriatr Psychiatry Neurol 9 (2): 53–6

20. Ortega RM, Lopez-Sobaler AM, Zamora MJ, Redondo R, Gonzalez-Gross M, Andres P (1996) Dietary intake of a physically active elderly Spanish male group of high socioeconomic status. Int J Food Sci Nutr 47 (4): 307–13

21. Perrig WJ, Perrig P, Stähelin HB (1997) The relation between antioxidants and memory performance in the old and very old. J Am Geriatr Soc 45 (6): 718–24

22. Rosenthal MJ, Goodwin JS (1985) Cognitive effects of nutritional deficiency. Adv Nutr Res 7 (71): 71–100

23. Smith MA, Monnier VM, Sayre LM, Perry G (1995) Amyloidosis, advanced glycation end products and Alzheimer disease [letter; comment]. Neuroreport 6 (12): 1595–6

24. Stähelin HB (1997) Antioxidants and atherosclerosis. In: Guesry P, Hennerici M, Sitzer G (eds) Nutrition and Stroke. Philadelphia: Lippincott-Raven. Nestlé Nutrition Workshop Series; Vol Supplement 1, pp 75–85

25. Wahlin A, Hill RD, Winblad B, Backman L (1996) Effects of serum vitamin B_{12} and folate status on episodic memory performance in very old age: a population-based study. Psychol Aging 11 (3): 487–96

Author's address:

Prof. Dr. med. Hannes B. Stähelin
Geriatrische Universitätsklinik
Kantonsspital
CH-4031 Basel, Switzerland
E-mail: staehelin1@ubaclu.unibas.ch

Undernutrition and osteoporosis

R. Rizzoli, J.-P. Bonjour

Division of Bone Diseases, World Health Organization Collaborating Center for Osteoporosis and Bone Diseases, Department of Internal Medicine, University Hospital, Geneva, Switzerland

Summary

Undernutrition, particularly protein undernutrition, contributes to the occurrence of osteoporotic fracture, by lowering bone mass and altering muscle strength. Furthermore, the rate of medical complications after fracture can also be increased by nutritional deficiency. The IGF-I system appears to be directly involved in the pathogenetic mechanisms leading to osteoporotic hip fracture in the elderly and to its complications. In the presence of adequate calcium and vitamin D supplies, protein supplements increasing the intakes from low to normal, raise IGF-I levels, improve the clinical outcome after hip fracture, and attenuate the decrease in proximal femur bone mineral density in the year following the fracture. This nutritional approach is associated with a significant reduction of the stay in rehabilitation hospital. This underlines the importance of nutritional supports in preventing and healing osteoporotic fractures.

Role of protein undernutrition in the occurrence of osteoporotic fracture

Osteoporosis, which is defined as a systemic skeletal disease characterized by low bone mass and microarchitectural deterioration of bone tissue, with a consequent increase in bone fragility and susceptibility to fracture (60), is widely recognized as a major problem of public health of the elderly. The number of fractures of the proximal femur, which represents the most dramatic expression of the disease, increases as the population ages (18, 49). A variety of different factors determine the risk of osteoporosis, including genetics, sex hormone deficiency, reduced physical exercise, and the influence of various environmental risk factors. Among the determinants of osteoporosis in the elderly, nutritional deficiencies certainly play a significant role (40, 48). Indeed, undernutrition is often observed in the elderly, and it appears to be more severe in patients with hip fracture than in the general aging population (8, 21, 32, 37, 44). Thus, deficiency in nutritional elements could play an important role in the pathogenesis of osteoporotic fracture in the elderly. Among the nutrients, many studies have indicated that calcium supplementation reduces bone loss and fracture incidence in vitamin D replete elderly subjects (15, 20).

Evidence also leads to the conclusion that protein intake far below the RDA could be particularly detrimental for both the acquisition of bone mass and the conservation of bone integrity with aging. Presently, the recommended daily allowance (RDA) for protein is age-dependent, since it varies between 2.0 in children to 1.0 in adolescents, and 0.75 g/kg body weight in adults (45). Protein undernutrition can favor the occurrence of hip fracture by increasing the propensity to fall as a result of muscle weakness and of impairment in movement coordination, by affecting protective mechanisms, such as reaction time, muscle strength, thus reducing the energy required to fracture an osteoporotic proximal femur (8), and/or by decreasing bone mass (25). Indeed, undernutrition could also accelerate age-dependent bone loss (24, 40, 48). Furthermore, a reduction in the protective layer of soft tissue padding decreases the force required to fracture an osteoporotic hip (26, 59).

A low plasma albumin level has been repeatedly found in patients with hip fracture as compared to age-matched healthy subjects or patients with osteoarthritis (21, 41, 44). In hip fracture patients, in whom a lower femoral neck BMD at the level of the proximal femur has been demonstrated (16), a dietary survey based on 50 daily precise measurements of food intake confirmed that nutritional requirements were not met while the patients were in hospital, although adequate quantities of food were offered (21). Various studies have found a relationship between the level of protein intake and calcium-phosphate or bone metabolism (4, 9, 19, 38) and have come to the conclusion that either a deficient or an excessive protein supply could negatively affect the balance of calcium. For instance, hip fracture appeared to be more frequent in countries with high protein intake of animal origin (1) but, as expected, the countries with the highest incidence are those with longest life expectancy, which could increase fracture incidence. In the large Nurse Health Study a trend for a hip fracture incidence inversely related to protein intake has been reported (22). Similarly, hip fracture was higher with low energy intake, low serum albumin levels, and low muscle strength in the NHANES I study (30). In a prospective study carried out on more than 40,000 women in Iowa, higher protein intake was associated with a reduced risk of hip fracture (35). Similarly, a reduced relative risk of hip fracture was found with higher intake of milk (33). In another survey, although no association between hip fracture and non-dairy animal protein intake could be detected, the fracture risk was increased when a high protein diet was accompanied by a low calcium intake (34). Regarding bone mineral mass results, there was a negative correlation with spontaneous protein intake in premenopausal women (19), and bone mineral mass was directly proportional to serum albumin in hip fracture patients (52). In a recent survey carried out in hospitalized elderly patients, low protein intake was associated with reduced femoral neck areal bone mineral density (BMD) and poor physical performances (25). The group with high intakes and a greater BMD, particularly at the femoral neck level, had also a better improvement of bicipital and quadricipital muscle strength and performance, as indicated by the increased capacity to walk and climb stairs, after four weeks of hospitalization (25). In a longitudinal follow-up in the frame of the Framingham study, the rate of bone mineral loss was inversely correlated to dietary protein intake (28). In contrast, in a cross-sectional study, a protein intake close to 2 g/kg body weight was associated with reduced bone mineral density only at one out of two forearm sites in young college women (4). Whereas a gradual decline in caloric intake with age can be considered as an adequate adjustment to the progressive reduction in energy expenditure, the parallel reduction in protein intake may be detrimental for maintaining the integrity and function of several organs or systems, including skeletal muscles and bone. In association with the progressive age-dependent decrease in both protein intake and bone mass, several reports have documented a decrement in IGF-I plasma levels (27, 43).

Nutritional control of insulin-like growth factor-I and bone homeostasis

Experimental and clinical studies suggest that dietary proteins, by influencing both the production and action of growth factors, particularly the Growth Hormone (GH) Insulin-like Growth Factor (IGF) system, could control bone anabolism (10, 46). The hepatic production and plasma level of IGF-I is under the influence of dietary proteins (31, 54). Protein restriction has been shown to reduce IGF-I plasma levels by inducing a resistance to the action of GH at the hepatic level (54, 55, 58) and by an increase of IGF-I metabolic clearance rate (53). Decreased levels of IGF-I have been found in states of undernutrition such as marasmus, anorexia nervosa, celiac disease or HIV infected patients (29, 42, 51, 54). Refeeding these patients led to an increase of IGF-I (17, 42). Furthermore, elevated protein intake is able to prevent the decrease in IGF-I usually observed in hypocaloric states (31, 36). In addition, protein restriction could render target systems less sensitive to IGF-I. When IGF-I was given to rats maintained under a low protein diet at doses normalizing their plasma levels, it failed to restore skeletal longitudinal growth (56).

IGF-I is an essential factor for longitudinal bone growth (23), as it stimulates proliferation and differentiation of chondrocytes in the epiphyseal plate (10). IGF-I also plays a role in trabecular and cortical bone formation. This factor can stimulate both proliferation and differentiation of osteoblasts; it increases type I collagen synthesis, alkaline phosphatase activity, and osteocalcin production. Furthermore, by its renal action on tubular reabsorption of phosphate and on the synthesis of calcitriol, through a direct action on renal cells (12, 13), IGF-I can be considered as an important controller of the intestinal absorption and of the extra-cellular concentration of both calcium and phosphate, the main elements of bone mineral. IGF-I can selectively stimulate the transport of inorganic phosphate across the plasma membrane in some osteoblastic cell lines (39).

Thus, we recently investigated the influence on BMD of IGF-I delivered by subcutaneous osmotic minipumps in adult rats made osteoporotic by ovariec-tomy. BMD was measured by dual energy X-ray absorptiometry at the levels of lumbar spine, proximal and total tibia. A 6-week infusion of IGF-I induced a dose-dependent increment of BMD at the three scanned skeletal sites (3). In this animal model the increase in BMD induced by IGF-I was not merely due to an increase in bone growth. It was associated with an increase in the resistance to mechanical strain in relation also with an increase of bone shaft outer dimensions (2, 3).

Osteogenic cells can not only be equipped with specific IGF-I receptors, but they can also be endowed with IGF-I producing machinery (10). Regarding a possible influence of the local environment in proteins or amino acids on IGF-I production by bone cells, it has been recently found that the amino acids arginine or lysine

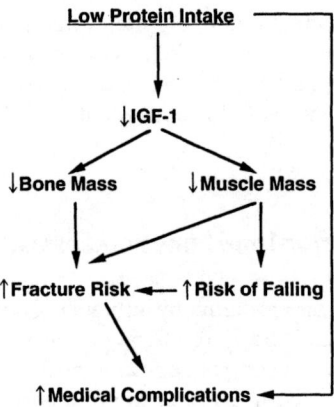

Fig. 1. Possible role of protein undernutrition and IGF-I in the pathogenesis of osteoporotic hip fracture and postfracture medical complications in elderly.

increased IGF-I production and collagen synthesis by a mice osteoblastic cell line in a time- and concentration-dependent manner (14). These results highlight the potential role of locally produced IGF-I under the influence of extracellular amino acid concentration in the regulation of osteoblast function.

Thus, IGF-I can exert anabolic effects on bone mass not only during growth, but also during adulthood. Taking into account these experimental and clinical observations, IGF-I could play a prominent role in the pathophysiology of osteoporosis, osteoporotic fracture, and its complications (Fig. 1). Under these conditions, a restoration of this altered system in elderly by protein replenishment is likely to favorably influence not only bone mineral density, but also muscle mass and strength since these two variables are important determinants (5, 11) of the risk of falling.

Outcome of fracture of the proximal femur

In accordance with several studies in which a state of undernutrition has been documented in elderly patients with hip fracture (7, 8, 32), several studies support the notion that a state of malnutrition on admission followed by an inadequate food intake during hospital stay can adversely influence the clinical outcome of elderly patients with hip fracture (7, 8, 2). The first evidence was obtained by intervention studies using supplementary feeding by nasogastric tube or parenteral nutrition (7). The clinical course of these patients could also be improved by providing a simple oral dietary preparation, since this way of correcting the deficient food intake has obvious practical and psychological advantages over nasogastric tube feeding or parenteral nutrition (21). In these patients, the clinical outcome after hip fracture was significantly improved by a daily oral nutritional supplement that normalized protein intake. It should be emphasized that a 20 g protein supplement brought the intake from low to a level still below the RDA, thus avoiding the risk of an excess of dietary protein. Clinical outcome was significantly better in the supplemented groups compared to the controls. Follow-up showed a significant

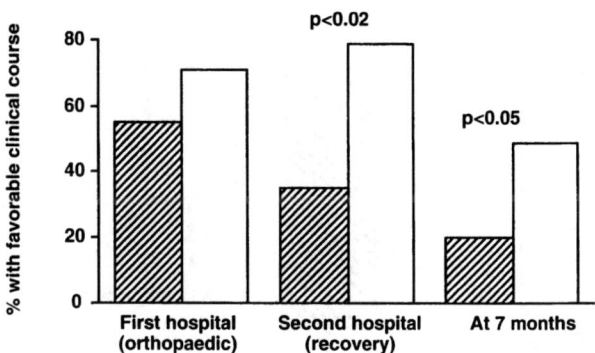

Fig. 2. Effects on medical complication rate of a milk protein daily supplement of 20 g in elderly with a recent hip fracture. Hashed bars: controls; dashed bars: protein supplemented patients. The results are taken from (57) with the permission of the publisher.

difference in the clinical course in the rehabilitation hospitals, with the supplemented patients doing better. Overall, 56 % of favorable course in the supplemented group as compared to 13 % in the controls was recorded. Although the mean duration of dietary supplementation did not exceed 30 d, the significantly lower rate of complication (bedsore, severe anemia, intercurrent lung or renal infections, 44 % vs 87 %) and deaths was still observed at six months (40 % vs 74 %) (21). The duration of hospital stay of elderly patients with hip fracture is not only determined by the actual medical condition, but also by domestic and social factors (7, 8, 49, 51). Nevertheless, in this study, the total length of stay in the orthopedic ward and convalescent hospital was significantly shorter in supplemented patients than in controls (median: 24 vs 40 d).

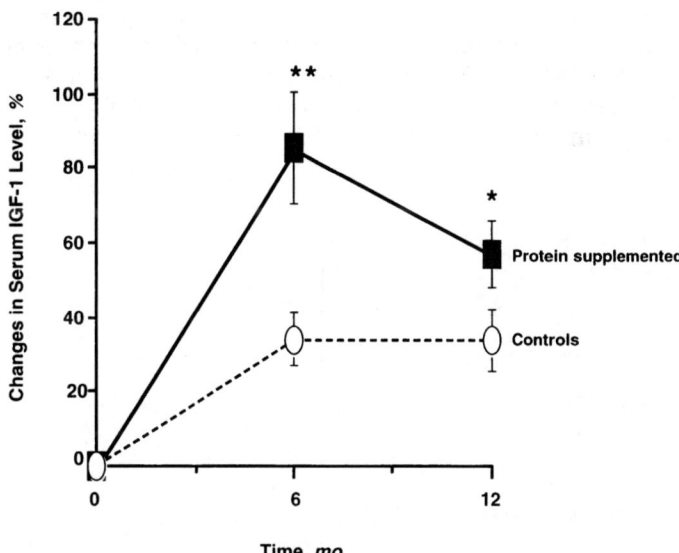

Fig. 3. Effects on serum IGF-I levels of a milk protein supplement of 20 g in elderly with a recent hip fracture; *p < 0.06; **p < 0.005. The results are taken from (50) with the permission of the publisher.

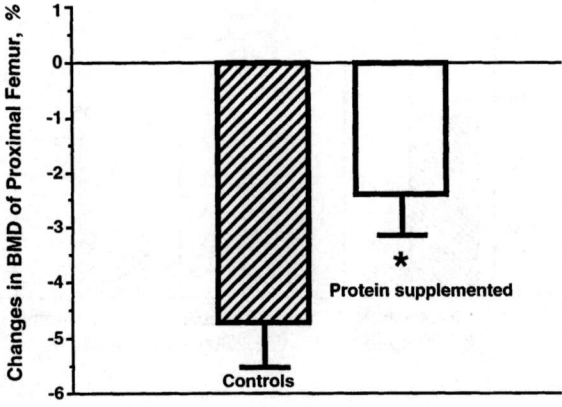

Fig. 4. Effects on proximal femur Bone Mineral Density of a daily milk protein supplement in elderly with a recent hip fracture; *p < 0.05. The results are adapted from (50) with the permission of the publisher.

In a subsequent study, it was shown that normalization of protein intake, independently of that of energy, calcium, and vitamin D, was in fact responsible for this more favorable outcome (57). Indeed, in addition to protein, various minerals and vitamins were also present in the supplement, as in previous reports using parenteral or nasogastric infusion (7). The question as to whether protein represented the key nutrient responsible for the beneficial effect was addressed by comparing the clinical outcome of elderly patients with hip fracture (mean age 82 years), receiving two different dietary supplements which only differed by their protein contents (57). The clinical course was significantly better in the group receiving protein, with 79 % having a favorable course, as compared to 36 % in the control group during the stay in the recovery hospital (Fig. 2).

In undernourished elderly with a recent hip fracture, an increase in the protein intake, from low to normal, can also be beneficial for bone integrity (50). Indeed, in a double-blind, placebo-controlled study, the effects of protein repletion were investigated in patients with a recent hip fracture. Within one week after an osteoporotic hip fracture, 82 patients (80.7 ± 1.2 yrs) were randomly allocated to a daily

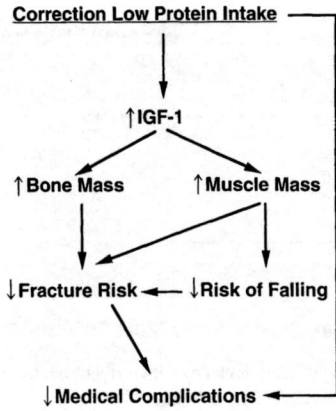

Fig. 5. Correction of protein undernutrition, risk of fracture, and outcome in elderly.

20 g protein supplement, which nearly corrected protein deficiency, or to an isocaloric placebo, for 6 months. All were given 200,000 IU vitamin D once at baseline, and 550 mg/d of calcium. In agreement with previous results (21, 57), protein repletion after hip fracture was associated with a more favorable outcome including a shorter rehabilitation hospital stay. In a multiple regression analysis, baseline IGF-I concentrations and biceps muscle strength, together with the presence of protein supplements, accounted for more than 30% of the variance of the length of stay in rehabilitation hopitals ($r^2 = 0.312, p < 0.0005$). As compared with the placebo group, the protein supplemented patients had significantly greater gains in serum prealbumin, IGF-I (Fig. 3), and IgM. In the protein supplemented patients, the proximal femur BMD decrease observed at one year in the placebo group was attenuated by approximately 50 % (Fig. 4). These results support the hypothesis that the beneficial effects of protein repletion after hip fracture could be associated with a stimulation of the IGF-I system (Fig. 5). The lower incidence of medical complications observed after such a supplement (21, 57) is also compatible with the hypothesis of IGF-I improving the immune status, as this growth factor can stimulate the proliferation of immunocompetent cells and modulate immunoglobulin secretion (6). These results raise the question whether protein repletion of frail elderly could prevent the age-dependent decrease in IGF-I levels, and help thereby to prevent falls and to increase bone mass. However, the effects of protein repletion in frail elderly at risk of osteoporotic fracture remain to be tested.

Acknowledgments   We thank Mrs. M. Perez for her secretarial assistance. The studies from our group quoted were supported by the Swiss National Research Foundation (Grants Nos. 32-32415.91 and 32-49957.96).

References

1. Abelow BJ, Holford TR, Insogna KL (1992) Cross-cultural association between dietary animal protein and hip fracture: a hypothesis. Calcif Tissue Int 50: 14–18
2. Ammann P, Rizzoli R, Meyer JM, Bonjour JP (1996) Bone density and shape as determinants of bone strength in IGF-I and/or pamidronate-treated ovariectomized rats. Osteoporos Int 6: 219–227
3. Ammann P, Rizzoli R, Muller K, Slosman D, Bonjour JP (1993) IGF-I and pamidronate increase bone mineral density in ovariectomized adult rats. Am J Physiol 265: E770–E776
4. Anderson JJB, Metz JA (1995) Adverse association of high protein intake to bone density. Challenges of Modern Medicine 7: 407–412
5. Aniansson A, Zetterberg C, Hedberg M, Henriksson K (1984) Impaired muscle function with aging. Clin Orthop 191: 193–201
6. Auernhammer CJ, Strasburger CJ (1995) Effects of growth hormone and insulin-like growth factor I on the immune system. Eur J Endocrinol 133: 635–645
7. Bastow MD, Rawlings J, Allison SP (1983) Benefits of supplementary tube feeding after fractured neck of femur: a randomised controlled trial. Br Med J 287: 1589–1592
8. Bastow MD, Rawlings J, Allison SP (1983) Undernutrition, hypothermia, and injury in elderly women with fractured femur: an injury response to altered metabolim? Lancet i: 143–146
9. Bonjour JP, Schürch MA, Rizzoli R (1996) Nutritional aspects of hip fractures. Bone 18 (Suppl 3): S139–144
10. Canalis E, McCarthy TL, Centrella M (1991) Growth factors and cytokines in bone cell metabolism. Annu Rev Med 42: 17–24

11. Castaneda C, Gordon PL, Fielding RA, Evans WJ, Crim MC (1997) Low-protein dietary intake results in reduced plasma IGF-I levels and skeletal muscle fiber atrophy in elderly women. Faseb J 11: abstr 1374

12. Caverzasio J, Bonjour JP (1989) Insulin-like growth factor I stimulates Na-dependent Pi transport in cultured kidney cells. Am J Physiol 257: F712–F717

13. Caverzasio J, Montessuit C, Bonjour JP (1990) Stimulatory effect of insulin-like growth factor-I on renal Pi transport and plasma 1,25-dihydroxyvitamin D3. Endocrinology 127: 453–459

14. Chevalley T, Rizzoli R, Manen D, Caverzasio J, Bonjour JP (1998) Arginine increases insulin-like growth factor-I production and collagen synthesis in osteoblast-like cells. Bone 23: 103–109

15. Chevalley T, Rizzoli R, Nydegger V, Slosman D, Rapin CH, Michel JP, Vasey H, Bonjour JP (1994) Effects of calcium supplements on femoral bone mineral density and vertebral fracture rate in vitamin D-replete elderly patients. Osteoporos Int 4: 245–252

16. Chevalley T, Rizzoli R, Nydegger V, Slosman D, Tkatch L, Rapin CH, Vasey H, Bonjour JP (1991) Preferential low bone mineral density of the femoral neck in patients with a recent fracture of the proximal femur. Osteoporos Int 1: 147–154

17. Clemmons DR, Underwood LE, Dickerson RN, Brown RO, Hak LJ, MacPhee RD, Heizer WD (1985) Use of plasma somatomedin-C/insulin-like growth factor-I measurements to monitor the response to nutritional repletion in malnourished patients. Am J Clin Nutr 41: 191–198

18. Cooper C, Melton III J (1992) Epidemiology of osteoporosis. Trends Endocrinol Metab 3: 224–229

19. Cooper C, Atkinson EJ, Hensrud DD, Wahner HW, O'Fallon WM, Riggs BL, Melton III LG (1996) Dietary protein intake and bone mass in women. Calcif Tissue Int 58: 320–325

20. Dawson-Hughes B, Harris SS, Krall EA, Dallal GE (1997) Effect of calcium and vitamin D supplementation on bone density in men and women 65 years of age or older. N Engl J Med 337: 670–676

21. Delmi M, Rapin CH, Bengoa JM, Delmas PD, Vasey H, Bonjour JP (1990) Dietary supplementation in elderly patients with fractured neck of the femur. Lancet i: 1013–1016

22. Feskanich D, Willett WC, Stampfer MJ, Colditz GA (1996) Protein consumption and bone fractures in women. Am J Epidemiol 143: 472–479

23. Froesch ER, Schmid C, Schwander J, Zapf J (1985) Actions of insulin-like growth factors. Annu Rev Physiol 47: 443–467

24. Garn SM, Guzman MA, Wagner B (1969) Subperiosteal gain and endosteal loss in protein-calorie malnutrition. Am J Phys Anthropol 30: 153–155

25. Geinoz G, Rapin CH, Rizzoli R, Kraemer R, Buchs B, Slosman D, Michel JP, Bonjour JP (1993) Relationship between bone mineral density and dietary intakes in the elderly. Osteoporos Int 3: 242–248

26. Grisso JA, Kelsey JL, Strom BL, Chiu GY, Maislin G, O'Brien LA, Hoffman S, Kaplan F and the Northeast Hip Fracture Study Group (1991) Risk factors for falls as a cause of hip fracture in women. N Engl J Med 324: 1326–1331

27. Hammerman MR (1987) Insulin-like growth factors and aging. Endocrinol Metab Clin North Am 16: 995–1011

28. Hannan MT, Tucker K, Dawson-Hughes B, Felson DT, Kiel DP (1997) Effect of dietary protein on bone loss in elderly men and women: the Framingham Osteoporosis Study. J Bone Miner Res 12 (Suppl 1): S151

29. Hill KK, Hill DB, McClain MP, Humphries LL, McClain CJ (1993) Serum insulin-like growth factor-I concentrations in the recovery of patients with anorexia nervosa. J Am Coll Nutr 4: 475–478

30. Huang Z, Himes JH, McGovern PG (1996) Nutrition and subsequent hip fracture risk among a national cohort of white women. Am J Epidemiol 144: 124–134

31. Isley WL, Underwood LE, Clemmons DR (1983) Dietary components that regulate serum somatomedin-C concentrations in humans. J Clin Invest 71: 175–182

32. Jensen JE, Jensen TG, Smith TK, Johnston DA, Dudrick SJ (1982) Nutrition in orthopaedic surgery. J Bone Joint Surg 64: 1263–1272

33. Johnell O, Gullberg B, Kanis JA, Allander E, Elffors L, Dequeker J, Dilsen G, Gennari C, Vaz AL, Lyritis G, Mazzuoli G, Miravet L, Passeri M, Cano RP, Rapado A, Ribot C (1995) Risk factors for hip fracture in European women: the MEDOS study. J Bone Miner Res 10: 1802–1815

34. Meyer HE, Pedersen JI, Løken EB, Tverdal A (1997) Dietary factors and the incidence of hip fracture in middle-aged Norwegians. A prospective study. Am J Epidemiol 145: 117–123

35. Munger RG, Cerhan J, Chiu B, Yang S, Allnutt K (1995) Protein intake and risk of hip fracture in a cohort of older IOWA women. Am Soc Clin Nutr Abstract

36. Musey VC, Goldstein S, Farmer PK, Moore PB, Phillips LS (1993) Differential regulation of IGF-I and IGF-binding protein-I by dietary composition in humans. Am J Med Sci 305: 131–138

37. Older MWJ, Edwards D, Dickerson JWT (1980) A nutrient survey in elderly women with femoral neck fractures. Br J Surg 67: 884–886

38. Orwoll ES (1992). The effects of dietary protein insufficiency and excess on skeletal health. Bone 13: 343–350

39. Palmer G, Bonjour JP, Caverzasio J (1996) Stimulation of inorganic phosphate transport by insulin-like growth factor I and vanadate in opossum kidney cells is mediated by distinct protein tyrosine phosphorylation processes. Endocrinology 137: 4699–4705

40. Parfitt AM (1983) Dietary risk factors for age-related bone loss and fractures. Lancet ii: 1181–1184

41. Patterson BM, Cornell CN, Carbone B, Levine B, Chapman D (1992) Protein depletion and metabolic stress in elderly patients who have a fracture of the hip. J Bone Joint Surg 74A: 251–260

42. Pucilowska JB, Davenport ML, Kabir I, Clemmons DR, Thissen JP, Butler T, Underwood LE (1993) The effect of dietary protein supplementation on insulin-like growth factors (IGFs) and IGF-binding proteins in children with shigellosis. J Clin Endocrinol Metab 77: 1516–1521

43. Quesada JM, Coopmans W, Ruiz B, Aljama P, Jans I, Bouillon R (1992) Influence of vitamin D on parathyroid function in the elderly. J Clin Endocrinol Metab 75: 494–501

44. Rapin CH, Lagier R, Boivin G, Jung A, MacGee W (1982) Biochemical findings in blood of aged patients with femoral neck fractures: a contribution to the detection of occult osteomalacia. Calcif Tissue Int 34: 465–469

45. Recommended Daily Allowances (1989) National Research Council (US), 10th edition. National Academy Press, Washington

46. Rosen CJ, Donahue LR (1995) Insulin-like growth factors: potential therapeutic options for osteoporosis. Trends Endocrinol. Metab 6: 235–241

47. Rosen C, Donahue LR, Hunter S, Holick M, Kavookjian H, Kirschenbaum A, Mohan S, Baylink DJ (1992) The 24/25-kDa serum insulin-like growth factor-binding protein is increased in elderly women with hip and spine fractures. J Clin Endocrinol Metab 74: 24–27

48. Schaafsma G, Van Beresteyn ECH, Raymakers JA, Duursma SA (1987) Nutritional aspects of osteoporosis. World Rev Nutr Diet 49: 121–159

49. Schürch MA, Rizzoli R, Mermillod B, Vasey H, Michel JP, Bonjour JP (1996) A prospective study on socioeconomic aspects of fracture of the proximal femur. J Bone Miner Res 11: 1935–1942

50. Schürch MA, Rizzoli R, Slosman D, Vadas L, Vergnaud P, Bonjour JP (1998) Protein supplements increase serum insulin-like growth factor-I levels and attenuate proximal femur bone loss in patients with recent hip fracture. A randomized, double-blind, placebo-controlled trial. Ann Intern Med 128: 801–809

51. Sullivan DH, Carter WJ (1994) Insulin-like growth factor I as an indicator of protein-energy undernutrition among metabolically stable hospitalized elderly. J Am Coll Nutr 13: 184–191

52. Thiébaud D, Burckhardt P, Costanza M, Sloutskis D, Gilliard D, Quinodoz F, Jacquet AF, Burnand B (1997) Importance of albumin, 25(OH)-vitamin D and IGFBP-3 as risk factors in elderly women and men with hip fracture. Osteoporos Int 7: 457–462

53. Thissen JP, Davenport ML, Pucilowska J, Miles MV, Underwood LE (1992) Increased serum clearance and degradation of (125I)-labeled IGF-I in protein-restricted rats. Am J Physiol 262: E406–E411

54. Thissen JP, Ketelslegers JM, Underwood LE (1994) Nutritional regulation of the insulin-like growth factors. Endocr Rev 15: 80–101
55. Thissen JP, Triest S, Moats-Statts BM, Underwood LE, Mauerhoff T, Maiter D, Ketelslegers JM (1991) Evidence that pretranslational and translational defects decrease serum IGF-I concentrations during dietary protein restriction. Endocrinology 129: 429–435
56. Thissen JP, Underwood LE, Maiter D, Maes M, Clemmons DR, Ketelslegers JM (1991) Failure of insulin-like growth factor-I (IGF-I) infusion to promote growth in protein-restricted rats despite normalization of serum IGF-I concentrations. Endocrinology 128: 885–890
57. Tkatch L, Rapin CH, Rizzoli R, Slosman D, Nydegger V, Vasey H, Bonjour JP (1992) Benefits of oral protein supplement in elderly patients with fracture of the proximal femur. J Am Coll Nutr 11: 519–525
58. VandeHaar MJ, Moats-Staats BM, Davenport ML, Walker JL, Ketelslegers JM, Sharma BK, Underwood LE (1991) Reduced serum concentrations of insulin-like growth factor-I (IGF-I) in protein-restricted growing rats are accompanied by reduced IGF-I mRNA levels in liver and skeletal muscle. J Endocrinol 130: 305–312
59. Vellas B, Baumgartner RN, Wayne SJ, Conceicao J, Lafont C, Albarede JL, Garry PJ (1992) Relationship between malnutrition and falls in the elderly. Nutrition 8: 105–108
60. WHO Technical Report Series (1994) Assessment of fracture risk and its application to screening for postmenopausal osteoporosis. Report of a WHO Study Group, 843, World Health Organization, Geneva

Author's address:

Prof. René Rizzoli, M.D.
Division of Bone Diseases
World Health Organization Collaborating Center for Osteoporosis and Bone Diseases
Department of Internal Medicine
University Hospital
1211 Geneva 14, Switzerland
E-mail: rizzoli@cmu.unige.ch

Causes of protein-energy malnutrition

D. R. Thomas

Division of Gerontology and Geriatric Medicine, Saint Louis University, St. Louis, MO, USA

Summary

In developed countries, medical conditions, rather than lack of food, are the main contributors to malnutrition. Undernutrition is especially common in older persons, occurring in 5–12 % of community-dwelling older persons, in 30–61 % of hospitalized older persons, and in 40–85 % of persons in long-term care institutions. The multi-factorial nature of undernutrition in the elderly forces a structured differential diagnostic approach to determine underlying causes. Heightened physician awareness of nutritional problems and prompt risk assessment is imperative to prevent the sequelae of undernutrition. This structured approach to the differential diagnosis is essential to evaluate potentially reversible causes of malnutrition.

Introduction

Worldwide, malnutrition is most often caused by lack of food. In developed countries, medical conditions, rather than lack of food, are the main contributors to malnutrition. Simple loss of appetite or anorexia is uncommon in healthy individuals, including the elderly. In anorexia, the failure to consume an adequate diet leads to classical signs and symptoms of malnutrition even when access to adequate food sources is intact.

Aging is associated with a lower energy intake. Almost one in five community-dwelling elderly persons consume less that 1,000 Kcal daily (1). On average, persons over the age of 70 years consume one third less calories compared to younger persons, with energy intake of older men (40–74 years old) in a range of 2100–2300 calories/d compared to younger men (24–34 years old) at 2700 calories/d (27).

Despite lower intake, the requirements for nearly all nutrients does not decline substantially with age (33). Nutrient requirements are expressed as a Recommended Dietary Allowance (RDA). Recommended Daily Allowances (RDA) are based on the minimal requirement for 95 % of the population based on a reference male, age 25, height 5'10", weight 150 pounds, with a normal body composition (14). There are no recommendations for persons older than 70 years due to higher prevalence of chronic disease, insufficient data, and heterogeneity of the population. Lower energy requirements were assumed for older persons and no adjustment was made for sex differences past age 51 (34).

Energy need determines total caloric food intake (10). Hallfrisch et al. (16) have shown a decline in total daily energy requirements after age 40. Daily energy requirements are made up of three distinct components: the resting energy expenditure (REE), the thermic effect of food, and the thermic effect of exercise (24). REE decreases with age, primarily due to a decrease in muscle mass. Active older adults have a higher REE than sedentary older adults (39), thus, reaching intakes equal of exceeding younger persons. Therefore, lower energy expenditure may be responsible for the observed lower energy intake in elderly persons.

Inadequate intake of macronutrients is termed protein-energy malnutrition. Malnutrition may result from inadequate protein intake relative to energy (kwashiorkor) or inadequate energy intake relative to protein (marasmus). Micronutrient intake of vitamins, mineral, and trace elements is closely linked to overall macronutrient intake. Although malnutrition includes overnutrition and undernutrition, this discussion is limited to undernutrition in older persons.

Prevalence of undernutrition

The prevalence of undernutrition is site-specific. Undernutrition reportedly occurs in 5–12 % of community-dwelling older persons, in 30–61 % of hospitalized older persons, and in 40–85 % of persons in long-term care institutions (46).

In community-dwelling persons, the prevalence of undernutrition depends on the methods used to define undernutrition. The largest estimated prevalence arises from dietary recall studies (26, 36). This results from comparing the recalled intake to the RDA standards. However, as energy intake declines with age, a decrease in the ratio of actual/recommended intake is inevitable. Despite lower energy intakes, the prevalence of biochemically measured inadequacies of macro- and micronutrient in community-dwelling older persons is quite low (9, 19, 54).

In hospitalized patients, nutritional status is poorly monitored status (22, 28, 40, 47) and patients often subsist on inadequate intake for days (41, 51). In this setting, severity of illness and other factors limit the patient's ability to consume an adequate diet. Nutritional status has been shown to deteriorate following hospital admission. When patients who had no current nutritional deficits and no predicted risk of developing deficits at hospital admission were followed, significant decreases in albumin, total lymphocyte count, tricep skinfold thickness, and mid-arm circumference occured in all patients by three weeks. The only nutritional parameter remaining unchanged at three weeks was percent of ideal body weight (38).

The highest prevalence for undernutrition is reported in long-term care. In nursing homes, the high prevalence of undernutrition may be related to medical conditions, anorexia, mechanical problems with consuming an adequate diet or inadequacies in nutritional management. Continued weight loss in long-term care facilities is common. In an academic nursing home, 60 % of residents experienced a net weight loss following admission (45). In a prospective study of institutionalized patients, there was a mean weight loss of 1.4 kg in the malnourished group while the normally nourished group gained a mean of 2.2 kg after admission (48).

Table 1 Risk factors for malnutrition

1. Social factors poverty, help with meals, shopping, lack of socialization
2. Mechanical barriers
   a. Poor oral health status or hygiene, eyesight, motor coordination, or taste alterations, such as rheumatoid arthritis or Parkinson's disease
   b. Slow eating pace resulting in food becoming unpalatable or in staff removing the tray before the resident has finished eating
   c. Failure to pay attention to ethnic preferences and lack of access to culturally acceptable foods
   d. Therapeutic or mechanically altered diet
3. Medical conditions
   a. Cancer
   b. Infections (acute and chronic)
   c. Hyperthyroidism and hyperparathyroidism
   d. Chronic obstructive pulmonary disease
   e. Congestive heart failure
   f. Malabsorption syndromes
   g. Diabetic gastroparesis
   h. Increased nutritional/caloric needs associated with pressure sores and wound healing (e.g. fractures, burns)
   i. AIDS
   j. Gall bladder disease
4. Psychiatric conditions
   a. Depression
   b. Dementia
   c. Late-life paranoia
   d. Anorexia nervosa

A structured diagnostic approach for undernutrition

The multi-factorial nature of undernutrition in the elderly forces a structured differential diagnostic approach to determine underlying causes. Table 1 lists common etiologies for undernutrition in the elderly. Using a series of questions for the differential diagnosis, the etiology of most causes of undernutrition can be determined (29).

Does the patient have access to food?

Social factors play a role in undernutrition in community settings. The extent to which these factors are responsible for undernutrition is poorly studied. Poverty, need for assistance with shopping or meal preparation, and lack of social incentives to consume an adequate diet have anecdotally been reported to cause undernutrition. Community meals, Meals-On-Wheels, and other social programs have been developed to counter these effects.

Can the patient eat?

The barriers to adequate intake must be assessed. These barriers are often overlooked, but represent potentially reversible conditions. Oral health factors may contribute to undernutrition. It is estimated that at least 80 % of nursing home residents have some degree of tooth loss, and that one third have mucosal lesions (50). Tooth loss has been strongly associated with undernutrition (37), but other investigators have questioned whether tooth loss affects nutritional status (5). Poor or ill-fitting dentures result in food avoidance (12). Data are inconclusive on the effect of new dentures on nutritional status (15). The ability to chew or swallow food may not correlate with the frequency of protein-energy malnutrition in institutional settings (48).

Dysphagia is a common problem in institutionalized persons. The causes can be neurologic, neuromuscular, or structural. Prescription medications may also cause swallowing dysfunction (4). Swallowing studies and mechanical alteration of diet often result in improved nutrition intake.

Does the patient have eye-hand coordination or muscular strength to self-feed?

Numerous medical conditions, such as stroke, Parkinson's disease, arthritis, neuropathies, and other neurological conditions, interfere with the ability to hold a utensil, raise the food to the mouth, or swallow. Adjustment of diet consistency or occupational therapy aids may ameliorate this difficulty.

Some patients must be assisted with feeding. A slow eating pace results in food becoming unpalatable, or in the caregiver removing the tray before the resident has finished eating. In demented institutionalized patients, an average of 18 min/d were spent in feeding compared to 99 min/d at home (18).

Assisting nursing home residents with eating is time and labor-intensive. Encouragement by the nursing staff to voluntary consume adequate calories is successful in very few residents (25). More intensive efforts to deliver calories to protein-energy malnourished residents may improve outcome. Further intervention studies need to be undertaken to determine if outcome can be improved by more aggressive feeding methods or the use of feeding teams to increase acceptance of diet (35).

Are there problems with the food?

Institutional food may be unpalatable. Many elderly nursing home residents grew up with poor dietary habits. The intake of eggs, cheese, ice cream, and liver may have been a life-long habit. Strong dietary preferences developed over a lifetime make adaptation to new foods problematic. Reductions in these types of foods may reduce quality-of-life perceptions in patients constrained to institutionalized diets. Similarly, failure to pay attention to the ethnic food preferences of the residents can result in food refusal and malnutrition.

The most common problem in institutional settings is an improper therapeutic or mechanically altered diet. Therapeutic diets themselves have also been shown to be associated with malnutrition in the nursing home (8, 32). The presence of co-morbid diseases frequently results in multiple dietary restrictions, including reduced salt intake, controlled calories, and carbohydrate restriction. The combination of institutional dietary restrictions may contribute to inadequate intake.

Since dietary fat is responsible for most food flavor, reductions in dietary fat can make food tasteless. Severe reductions in saturated fats may make diets monotonous. The net effect of reductions in dietary fat, combined with alterations in taste due to aging or drugs may result in inadequate food intake. Reductions in dietary fat intake influences of other nutrients. For example, decreasing saturated fat intake may result in inadequate calcium intake. About 60 % of daily calcium intake is derived from dairy products. Substitutes for these dairy products may not be acceptable to elderly patients.

Complicating dietary restriction is the fact that dietary therapy is often ineffective. Dietary reductions in fats may only reduce elevated cholesterol by 10–15 %. A minority of hypertensive patients are salt-sensitive. Liberalizing dietary prescriptions may avoid inadequate nutritional intake.

Does the patient have a medical condition that increases protein-energy requirements?

Cancer is the single largest identifiable reason for weight loss due to increased metabolic need in older persons (49). Cachectin has been implicated in the anorexia occurring with cancer (53). Although cancer represents the largest category of weight loss, less than 20 % of all weight loss is due to cancer. Undiagnosed cancer must be considered in patients who are losing weight, but is rarely found to be the cause. In patients with known cancer, provision of adequate calories is obvious. Nevertheless, cancer cachexia is resistant to correction with increased nutrition (52).

Infections, both acute and chronic, are an important cause of malnutrition occuring in 15–20 % of nursing home residents (43). Infection can result in confusion, anorexia, and negative nitrogen balance all of which may contribute to malnutrition (6). Acquired immunodeficiency syndrome (AIDS), frequently associated with weight loss and undernutrition (55), is not rare in elderly populations.

A number of other medical conditions contribute to undernutrition. Apathetic hypothyroidism may be associated with weight loss and difficult to diagnose. Chronic obstructive pulmonary disease is associated with increased energy needs due to increased work of breathing. Congestive heart failure is associated with weight loss. Malabsorption syndromes may cause weight loss due to poor use of

Table 2 Clinical conditions demonstrating that the maintenance of acceptable nutritional status may not be possible

1. Prolonged nausea, vomiting, diarrhea not relieved by treatment given according to accepted standards of practice
2. Refusal to eat and refusal of other methods of nourishment
3. Advanced disease (i.e., cancer, malabsorption syndrome)
4. Increased nutritional/caloric needs associated with pressure sores and wound healing (e.g. fractures, burns)
5. Radiation or chemotherapy
6. Chronic renal failure
7. Alcohol/drug abuse
8. Chronic gastrointestinal blood loos
9. Hyperthyroidism
10. Gastrointestinal surgery

foods presented to the gastrointestinal tract. Increased metabolic needs for tissue repair can occur in patients with pressure ulcers, burns, and fractures. Parkinson's disease and rheumatoid arthritis may induce malnutrition and weight loss by causing hypermetabolism, anorexia, swallowing difficulty, and/or malabsorption. Elevated levels of circulating cytokines, resulting in increased resting energy expenditure and decreased serum albumin level, have been implicated as a possible mechanism of malnutrition in conditions such as rheumatoid arthritis, chronic infections, and AIDS (17, 42).

Does the patient have a medical condition that interfere with eating?

Prolonged nausea, vomiting, or diarrhea may result in inadequate intake. Conditions commonly associated with nausea include radiation or chemotherapy, diabetic gastroparesis leading to delayed gastric emptying, gastrointestinal surgery, chronic renal failure, chronic gastrointestinal blood loss, alcohol/drug abuse, and gall bladder disease. These conditions may be difficult to relieve even when treated according to accepted standards of practice. Table 2 lists causes of malnutrition which may be poorly responsive to nutritional interventions.

Does the patient have anorexia?

Anorexia may result from the physiological changes of aging. A decrease in energy intake, as noted above, may result from decreased energy expenditure. Anorexia may result from a decrease in taste or smell. The number of taste receptors on the tongue decrease with aging (3), but the effect on nutrient intake is controversial (21). Smell dramatically decreases with age, and reduces the ability to correctly recognize foods (44). A number of medications also affect taste and smell (2).

One of the most common and potentially reversible causes of anorexia is related to adverse drug effects. Medications can induce undernutrition not only by causing anorexia, but also by inducing nausea, vomiting, diarrhea, constipation, cognitive

Table 3 Drug therapy that may contribute to nutritional deficiencies

A. cardiac glycosides
B. diuretics
C. anti-inflammatory drugs
D. antacids (overuse)
E. H2 blockers (cimetidine)
F. psychotropic drug overuse
G. antidepressants (serotonin-reuptake inhibitors)
H. anticonvulsants
I. antineoplastic drugs
J. phenothiazine
K. oral hypoglycemics

disturbance, or increased metabolism (29). The medications most frequently implicated include digoxin, theophylline, nonsteroidal anti-inflammatory drugs, iron supplements, and psychotropic drugs particularly fluoxetine, lithium, and phenothiazines. Table 3 lists common categories of drugs that contribute to nutritional problems.

Undernutrition itself may produce anorexia, the so-called terminal anorexia of malnutrition. A malabsorption syndrome associated with severe malnutrition may interfere with refeeding. Zinc deficiency has been shown to decrease feeding in animals, although not in humans (11).

Neurotransmitter regulators of food intake have been implicated in anorexia of aging. Gastrointestinal hormones, including cholecystokinin, gastrin releasing peptide, and somatostatin, and bombesin regulate satiety in humans to varying degrees (30). The importance of these neurotransmitters in part lies in the effect of certain classes of neuroactive antidepressant medications to either stimulate or suppress appetite.

Are there psychological problems that decrease intake?

Depression is one of the most common reversible causes of weight loss in the nursing home. Weight loss affects 8–38 % of nursing home residents (13). An analysis of 6832 Minimum Data Sets from 202 nursing homes in seven states showed that depression was associated with weight loss (7). Morley et al. (29) found depression to be the most common cause of weight loss in nursing home residents. Similarly, Katz et al. (23) reported that "failure to thrive" in nursing home residents was closely correlated with depression. Treatment of depression has been shown to result in weight gain (20). Proper recognition of depression may lead to a reverse of undernutrition.

Dementia is commonly associated with malnutrition, particularly in nursing home settings. In most cases this is due to the inability of demented residents to recognize the need to eat. Excessive wandering, psychotropic medications, paranoid ideation, the frequently associated depression, and the insufficient time spent on feeding because of inadequate staff are other factors that may contribute to malnutrition in residents with dementia. Some residents with dementia develop apraxia of swallowing and need to be reminded to swallow after each mouthful of food (31). While there is a generally held belief that patients with Alzheimer's disease have an increased metabolism, scientific evidence for this is lacking.

Table 4 Meals-on-wheels pneumonic for malnutrition

Medications	Oral factors	Wandering (dementia)
Emotional problems (depression)	No money	Hyperthyroidism, hyperparathyroidism, hypoadrenalism
Anorexia		Enteric problems (malsborption)
Late-life paranoia		Eating problems (inability to self-feed)
Swallowing disorders		Low-salt, low cholesterol diet
		Social problems

From: Morley JE, Silver AJ (1995) Nutritional issues in nursing home care. Ann Intern Med 123: 850–859

Late-life paranoia, late-life mania, and anorexia nervosa are other psychiatric conditions that may cause undernutrition. Anorexia nervosa is uncommon in elderly persons, but often misdiagnosed.

Conclusions

The causes of undernutrition in elderly persons is multi-factorial. Heightened physician awareness of nutritional problems and prompt risk assessment is imperative to prevent the sequelae of undernutrition. A structured approach to the differential diagnosis is essential to evaluate potentially reversible causes. A pneumonic useful in recalling the categories of undernutrition causes is shown in Table 4.

References

1. Abraham S, Carroll MD, Dresser CM et al. (1977) Dietary intake of persons 1–74 years of age in the United States. Advance Data from Vital and Health Statistics of the National Center for Health Statistics No. G, Rockville, MD, Public Health Service, March
2. Allara E (1939) Investigations on the human taste organ. Arch Ital Anat Embriol 42: 506–514
3. Arey LB, Tremaine MJ, Monzinga FL (1936) The numerical and topographical relations of taste buds to human circumvallate papillae throughout the live span. Anat Rec Suppl 64: 9–25
4. Baum BJ, Bodner L (1986) Aging and oral motor function: evidence for altered performance among older persons. Spec Care Dent 6: 80–83
5. Baxter JC (1984) The nutritional intake of geriatric patients with varied dentition. J Prosthet Dent 51: 164–168
6. Beisel WR (1977) Magnitude of the host nutritional responses to infection. Am J Clin Nutr 30: 1236–1247
7. Blaum CS, Fries BE, Fiatarone MA (1995) Factors associated with low body mass index and weight loss in nursing home residents. J Gerontol 50: M162–8
8. Buckler DA, Kelber ST, Goodwin JS (1994) The use of dietary restrictions in malnourished nursing home patients. J Am Geriatr Soc 42: 1100–1102
9. Burns R, Nichols L (1986) Nutritional assessment of community living elderly. J Am Geriatr Soc 34: 781–786
10. Durnin JVGA (1985) Energy intake, energy expenditure, and body composition in the elderly. In: Chandra RK (ed) Nutrition, immunity and illness in the elderly. Pergamon, New York, pp 19–33
11. Essatara MB, Levine AS, Morley JE et al. (1984) Zinc deficiency and anorexia in rates: normal feeding patterns and stress-induced feeding. Physiol Behav 32: 2793
12. Ettinger RL (1973) Diet, nutrition, and masticatory ability in a group of elderly edentulous patients. Aust Dent J 18: 12–19
13. Fitten LJ, Morley JE, Gross PI, Petry SD, Cole KD (1989) Depression. J Am Geriatric Soc 37: 459–72
14. Food and Nutrition Board, National Research Council (1990) Recommended dietary allowances. 10th edition. Washington, DC, National Academy Press
15. Gunne HS, Wall AK (1985) The effect of new complete dentures on mastication and dietary intake. Acta Odontol Scand 43: 257–268
16. Hallfrisch J, Muller D, Drinkwater D, Tobin J, Andres R (1990) Continuing diet rends in men: The Baltimore Longitudinal Study of Aging (1961–1987). J Gerontol 45: M186–191
17. Hellerstein MK, Kahn J, Mudie H et al. (1990) Current approach to the treatment of human immunodeficiency virus-associated weight loss: pathologic considerations and emerging management strategies. Semin Oncol 17 (Suppl 9): 17–33

18. Hu T, Huang L, Cartwright WS (1986) Evaluation of the costs of caring for the senile demented elderly: a pilot study. Gerontologist 26: 158–163
19. Jernigan JA, Gudat JC (1980) Reference values for blood findings in relatively fit elderly persons. J Am Geriatr Soc 28: 308–314
20. Kahn R (1995) Weight loss and depression in a community nursing home. J Am Geriatr Soc 43: 83
21. Kamath SK (1982) Taste acuity and aging. Am J Clin Nutr 36: 766–775
22. Kamath SK, Lawler M, Smith AE et al. (1986) Hospital malnutrition: A 33-hospital screening study. J Am Diet Assoc 86: 203–206
23. Katz IR, Beaston-Wimmer P, Parmetee P, Friedman E, Lawton MP (1993) Failure to thrive in the elderly: exploration of the concept and delineation of psychiatric components. J Geriatr Psychiatry Neurol 6: 151–69
24. Kendrick ZV, Nelson-Steen S, Scafidi K (1994) Exercise, aging, and nutrition. Southern Med J 87: S50–60
25. Lipschitz DA (1982) Protein calorie malnutrition in the hospitalized elderly. Primary care 9: 531–543
26. McGandy RB, Russell RM, Hartz SC, Jacob RA, Tannenbaum S, Peters H, Sahyoun N, Otradovec CL (1986) Nutritional status survey of healthy noninstitutionalized elderly: energy and nutrient intakes from three-day diet records and nutrient supplements. Nutr Res 6: 785–798
27. McGandy RB, Barrows CH Jr, Spanias A, Meredity A, Stone JL, Norris AH (1966) Nutrient intake and energy expenditure in men of different ages. J Gerontol 21: 581–587
28. McNab H, Restivo R, Ber L et al. (1987) Dietetic quality assurance practices in Chicago area hospitals. J Am Diet Assoc 85: 635–637
29. Morley JE, Kraenzie D (1994) Causes of weight loss in a community nursing home. J Am Geriatr Soc 42: 583–585
30. Morley JE, Silver AJ (1988) Anorexia in the elderly. Neurobiology of Aging 9: 9–16
31. Morley JE (1996) Anorexia in older persons. Drugs Aging 8 (2): 134–152
32. Morley JE, Kraenzle DK, Jensen JM, Gettman J, Tetter L (1994) The role of a nurse practitioner in quality improvement in nursing homes. Nursing Home Med 2: 11–19
33. Munro HN, Suter PM, Russel RM (1987) Nutritional requirements of the elderly. Ann Rev Nutrition 7: 23–49
34. Munro HN, Suter PM, Russel RM (1987) Nutritional requirements of the elderly. Ann Rev Nutrition 7: 23–49
35. Musson ND, Kincaid J, Ryan P, Glussman B, Varone L, Gamarra N, Wilson R, Reefe W, Silverman M (1990) Nature, nurture, nutrition: interdisciplinary programs to address the prevention of malnutrition and dehydration. Dysphagia 5 (2): 96–101
36. National Center for Health Statistics (1974) First health and nutrition examination survey, United States, 1971–1982, DHEW Publ No 74: 1219–1. Health Services Administration, Washington, DC
37. Neill DJ, Phillips HI (1972) The masticatory performance and dietary intake of elderly edentulous patients. Dent Pract 22: 384–389
38. Pinchcofsky GD, Kaminski MV Jr (1985) Increasing malnutrition during hospitalization: Documentation by a nutritional screening program. J Am Coll Nutri 4: 471–479
39. Poehlman ET, McAuliffe TL, Van Houten DR et al. (1990) Influence of age and endurance training on metabolic rate and hormones in healthy men. Am J Physiol 259: E66–72
40. Prevost EA, Butterworth CE (1974) Nutritional care of hospitalized patients. Am J Clin Nutr 27: 432
41. Riffer J (1986) Malnourished patients feeding rising costs. Hospitals 60: 86
42. Roubenoff R, Roubenoff RA, Cannon JG (1994) Rheumatoid cachexia: cytokine driven hypermetabolism and loss of lean body mass in chronic inflammation. J Clin Invest 93: 2379–86
43. Rudman D, Feller AG (1989) Protein-calorie undernutrition in the nursing home. J Am Geriatric Soc 37: 173–183
44. Schiffman S (1977) Food recognition by the elderly. J Gerontol 32: 586–592

45. Silver AJ, Morley JE, Strome LS, Jones D, Vickers L (1988) Nutritional status in an academic nursing home. J Am Geriatr Soc 36: 487–491
46. Silver AJ (1991) Malnutrition. In: Beck JC (ed) Geriatrics review syllabus. A core curriculum in geriatric medicine. Book 1/syllabus and questions. New York: American Geriatrics Society
47. Sullivan DH, Moriarty MS, Chernoff R et al. (1989) Patterns of care: an analysis of the quality of nutritional care routinely provided to elderly hospitalized veterans. JPEN 13: 249–254
48. Thomas DR, Verdery RB, Gardner L, Kant A, Lindsay J (1991) A prospective study of outcome from protein-energy malnutrition in nursing home residents. JPEN 15: 400–404
49. Thompson MP, Morris LK (1991) Unexplained weight loss in the ambulatory elderly. J Am Geriatr Soc 39: 497–500
50. Thomson WM, Brown RH, Williams SM (1992) Dentures, prosthestic treatment needs, and mucosal health in institutionalized elderly population. N Z Dent J 88: 51–5
51. Tobias AL, Van Itallie TB (1977) Nutritional problems of hospitalized patients. J Am Diet Assoc 71: 253–257
52. von Meyenfeldt MR, Fredrix EW, Haagh WA, van der Aalst AC, Soeters PB (1988) The aetiology and management of weight loss and malnutrition in cancer patients. Baillieres Clinical Gastro 2: 869–885
53. Wei H, Tracey K, Manogue K, Nguyen H, Fong Y, Hesse D, Beutler B, Solomon R, Cerami A, Lowry S (1987) Cachectin mediates suppressed food intake and anemia during chronic administration. Fed Proc 46: 1339A
54. Yearick ES, Wang MS, Pisias SJ (1980) Nutritional status of the elderly: dietary and biochemical findings. J Gerontol 35: 663–671
55. Zangerle R, Reibnegger G, Wachter H, Fuchs D (1993) Weight loss in HIV-1 infection is associated with immune activation. AIDS 7 (2): 175–81

Author's address:

David R. Thomas, MD, FACP
Professor of Medicine
Division of Geriatric Medicine
1402 South Grand Blvd., M238
St. Louis, MO 63104, USA

Nutritional evaluation tools in the elderly*

S. Lauque, F. Nourhashemi, B. Vellas

Department of Internal Medicine and Clinical Gerontology (Prof. JL Albarède), Toulouse, France

Summary

Malnutrition is frequent in the elderly, especially if frail or hospitalized. Nutritional evaluation tools allow the early detection of malnutrition and should be incorporated into the standard gerontological work-up as a basis for preventive action or rapid appropriate intervention. We review the various nutritional evaluation tools available, in particular the Mini Nutritional Assessment (MNA) which both evaluates nutritional status and guides nutritional intervention.

Introduction

Standard gerontological work-up of overall health status in the elderly employs simple, rapid, inexpensive and internationally validated scales for rating cognitive function, functional status, walking, balance, and socioeconomic status. Resulting corrective intervention helps to lower mortality, improve quality of life, and save healthcare costs (30, 33). The standard work-up should also incorporate nutritional status rating since not only is malnutrition a prognostic factor closely related to mortality and morbidity but its prevalence, which is relatively low in free-living elderly (5–10 %), rises considerably (30–60 %) in hospitalized or institutionalized elderly (1).

Conventional malnutrition assessment comprising anthropometrics, dietary recall, and laboratory investigation is too long and expensive as a first-line strategy. A number of simple rapid tests for detecting and/or diagnosing malnutrition in the elderly have recently been developed and in some cases validated (Table 1). Nutrition screening (27) involves identifying the characteristics associated with nutritional problems in the general population. The aim is to detect the subjects at risk from malnutrition, identify the cause(s), and guide corrective action. If malnourishment is suspected, these tests are supplemented by conventional nutritional assessment before planning treatment. These standard tests are also used in the overall work-up for diagnosing malnutrition states in combination with the medical and nutritional history, medical treatments, clinical examination, anthropometric measures, and laboratory results.

---

* This contribution was translated from French to English by Charles Kreeger MD and Ian Young MD, Lingua Medica, 51 Bartholomew Close (2nd floor), St. Bartholomew's Hospital, London EC1A 7BE, Email: BartsBiomedical@compuserve.com

Table 1. Nutritional evaluation tools: summary table

	NRS	NSI	Payette	SCALES	NRI	PNI	SGA	MNA	NuRAS
Sensitivity (%)		36	78		46	93	82	96	
Specificity (%)		85	77		85	44	72	98	
Cost	+	+	+	+++	+	+++	++	+	+
Time	Quick	Quick	Quick	Slow	Quick	Slow	Inter-mediate*	Quick	Quick
Type of elderly	At home	At home	Frail	Ill	At home	Ill	Ill	All	At home
Detects malnutrition?	Yes	Yes	Yes	No	Yes	No	No	Yes	Yes
Diagnoses malnutrition?	No	No	No	Yes	No	Yes	Yes	Yes	No
Nutritional follow-up	No	No	No	No	No	No	No	Yes	No

*	patient requires to be undressed
+	cheap
++	fairly expensive due to the requirement for a healthcare professional
+++	expensive due to laboratory investigations
MNA	Mini Nutritional Assessment
NRI	Nutrition Risk Index
NRS	Nutrition Risk score
NSI	Nutrition Screening Initiative
Nuras	Nutrition Risk Assessment Scale
PNI	Prognostic Nutritional Index
SGA	Subjective Global Assessment

Nutritional evaluation tools

Mini nutritional assessment

The mini nutritional assessment (MNA) (Fig. 1) (13, 14) is an 18-item nutritional questionnaire for the elderly developed and validated jointly by the Center for Internal Medicine and Clinical Gerontology of Toulouse (France), the Clinical Nutrition Program at the University of New Mexico (USA), and the Nestlé Research Center in Lausanne (Switzerland). It was validated in a total of 600 elderly of varying health status (free-living, at-risk, and institutionalized) after first being developed in Toulouse in 1991, then further validated in 1993. It was also tested in Albuquerque (New Mexico) in free-living elderly sharing a cultural context different from that in Toulouse and who had been participating in a longitudinal study started over 15 years previously. Since their nutritional status was fully documented, they were the ideal population for validating the test. The MNA was compared to a gold standard defined as the opinion of two nutritional physicians with access to the results of full nutritional assessment comprising laboratory results, anthropometrics, body weight, dietary recall, and the complete medical records. Good correlations were found with plasma albumin and prealbumin. The items comprise:

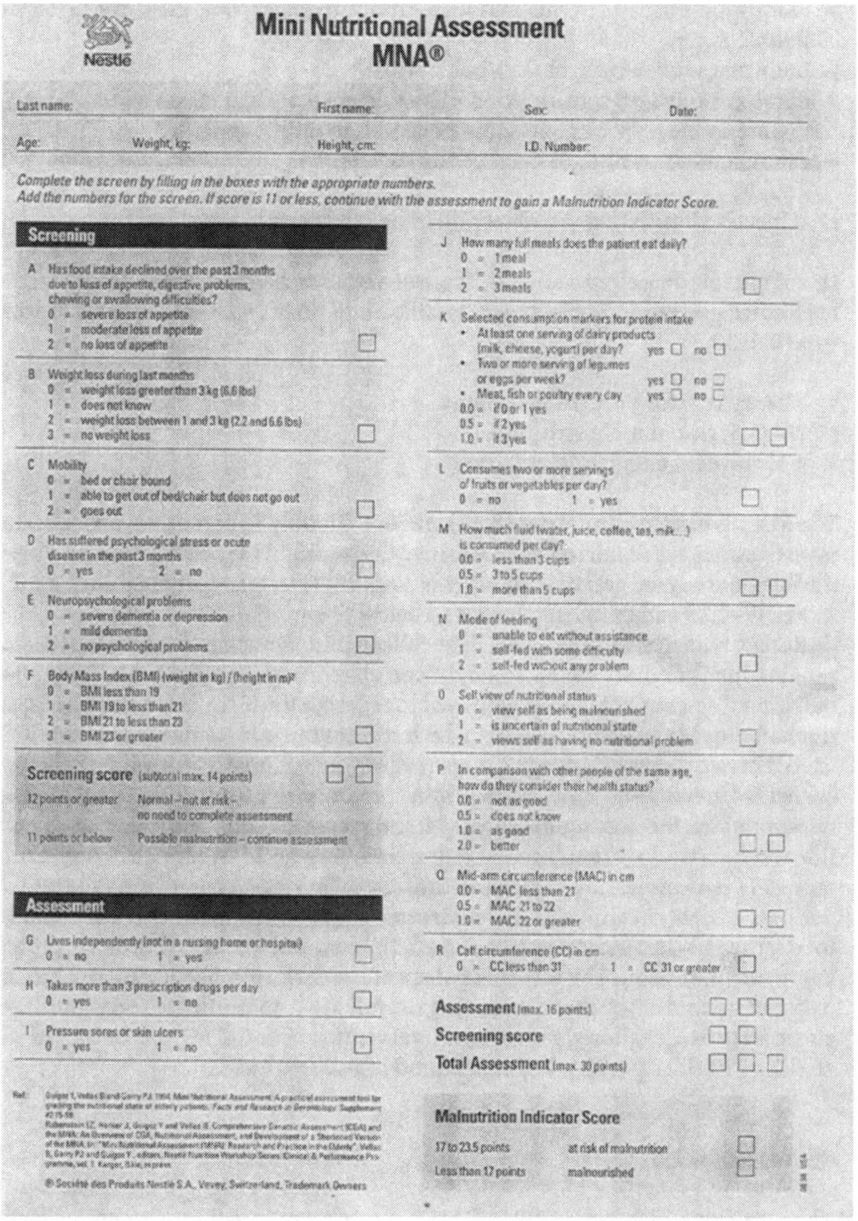

Fig. 1. Mini Nutritional Assessment (MNA®).

▶ anthropometrics (4) (calf and arm circumference) as a measure of fat and muscle mass;
▶ body mass index [weight (kg)/height (m)²];
▶ number of drugs (consumption of > 3 drugs daily can cause anorexia), acute disease in the previous 3 months, bedsores, mobility, appetite;
▶ eating habits: number of meals, daily consumption of protein, vegetables, fruit, liquids;
▶ subjective health (a good reflection of health status in the elderly).

In cognitively impaired subjects, the test requires help from the family and/or healthcare personnel. Subjects are classified into three levels on the basis of scores from 0 to 30:

▶ ≥ 24: satisfactory nutritional status
▶ 17–23.5: risk of malnutrition
▶ < 17: protein energy malnutrition.

The MNA is easy to administer (8, 11), patient-friendly, inexpensive (no laboratory investigations are required), very sensitive (96 %), highly specific (98 %), and reproducible: a study in geriatric inpatients found interrater reproducibility good at scores 17–23.5 and excellent above and below this range (10).

Recent reanalysis of the MNA data collected in Toulouse (France) and Mataro (Spain) identified six items strongly correlated with conventional (physician) nutritional assessment. These were used to redesign the MNA into a validated questionnaire for use in healthy elderly which still contains 18 items but is now administered in two stages (25). Stage 1 is a screening questionnaire using the six strongly correlated items (Fig. 1). It takes 3 min to administer vs 10 min for the overall questionnaire; the maximum score is 14, and scores ≥ 12 indicate satisfactory nutritional status, with no requirement to proceed to stage 2 (assessment). A screening score ≤ 11 is an indication to proceed to assessment stage 2, comprising the remainder of the MNA, in which case the screening and assessment scores are totalled: total scores 17–23.5 indicate a risk of malnutrition, and scores < 17 indicate protein-energy malnutrition. The screening stage of the MNA can be viewed as a preliminary nutritional assessment, reserving the full MNA to confirm the diagnosis and above all to guide tailored nutritional intervention. The full MNA is best used with at-risk or ill elderly with a high likelihood of malnutrition.

Nutritional risk index

The nutritional risk index (NRI) (22, 37) is a 16-item questionnaire on the factors impacting eating behavior: diet, dentition, gastrointestinal disorders, change in diet, etc. It separates subjects into two categories: satisfactory/unsatisfactory nutritional status. The questionnaire is easily administered by any healthcare professional, including over the telephone, and does not require preliminary training.

Nutrition risk score

The nutrition risk score (NRS) (15) is a validated tool for assessing malnutrition risk in free-living elderly using five categories of questions on body weight, body mass index, appetite, mode of feeding (self-feeding, mastication, vomiting, diarrhea, dysphagia, etc.), recent diseases, and surgical operations. Patients are classified as being at low, moderate or high risk; advice is given for each category.

The Warning Signs of poor nutritional health are often overlooked. Use this checklist to find out if you or someone you know is at nutritional risk.

Read the statements below. Circle the number in the yes column for those that apply to you or someone you know. For each yes answer, score the number in the box. Total your nutritional score.

DETERMINE YOUR NUTRITIONAL HEALTH

	YES
I have an illness or condition that made me change the kind and/or amount of food I eat.	2
I eat fewer than 2 meals per day.	3
I eat few fruits or vegetables, or milk products.	2
I have 3 or more drinks of beer, liquor or wine almost every day.	2
I have tooth or mouth problems that make it hard for me to eat.	2
I don't always have enough money to buy the food I need.	4
I eat alone most of the time.	1
I take 3 or more different prescribed or over-the-counter drugs a day.	1
Without wanting to, I have lost or gained 10 pounds in the last 6 months.	2
I am not always physically able to shop, cook and/or feed myself.	2
TOTAL	

Total Your Nutritional Score. If it's —

0-2 **Good!** Recheck your nutritional score in 6 months.

3-5 **You are at moderate nutritional risk.** See what can be done to improve your eating habits and lifestyle. Your office on aging, senior nutrition program, senior citizens center or health department can help. Recheck your nutritional score in 3 months.

6 or more **You are at high nutritional risk.** Bring this checklist the next time you see your doctor, dietitian or other qualified health or social service professional. Talk with them about any problems you may have. Ask for help to improve your nutritional health.

These materials developed and distributed by the Nutrition Screening Initiative, a project of:

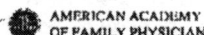 AMERICAN ACADEMY OF FAMILY PHYSICIANS

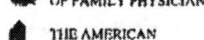 THE AMERICAN DIETETIC ASSOCIATION

NATIONAL COUNCIL ON THE AGING, INC.

Remember that warning signs suggest risk, but do not represent diagnosis of any condition. Turn the page to learn more about the Warning Signs of poor nutritional health.

Fig. 2. Nutrition Screening Initiative (NSI) (35).

Nutrition screening initiative

The nutrition screening initiative (NSI) (9, 35) is a multidisciplinary American undertaking to raise awareness of malnutrition risk among the elderly. Individuals or their carers can identify and correct risk factors for malnutrition using a questionnaire (Fig. 2). If the replies indicate poor nutritional status, the individual requires assessment at two levels. Level 1 assessment is performed by a healthcare professional (dietician, nurse, or doctor) and consists of body weight, body mass index, inquiry as to changes in weight, eating habits, place of residence, and performance status. Level 1 separates the elderly into two categories: those with a significant change in body weight requiring referral to a physician for level 2 assessment and those with less marked nutritional deficit requiring preventive intervention (nutritional information, meals on wheels, etc.). However, the elderly are often ignorant of their baseline body weight, in particular the at-risk individuals who rarely weigh themselves and are at greatest risk of malnutrition. Level 2 assessment by the physician comprises anthropometrics, plasma albumin and cholesterol, assessment of cognitive function, emotional and functional status, number of drugs, social setting, and clinical signs of malnutrition. The NSI is, therefore, designed to sensitize elderly to the situations that can give rise to malnutrition and provide them with means to respond with medical social worker aid. The test has only been validated against 24 h dietary recall.

Nutrition risk assessment scale

The nutrition risk assessment scale (NuRAS) is a validated 12-item questionnaire (20) assessing malnutrition risk factors in the elderly from data on gastrointestinal disorders, painful chronic disease, mobility, decrease in body weight and appetite, difficulty in eating, cognitive function, use of drugs, alcohol and tobacco, and social situation. The maximum score of 12 indicates a high risk of malnutrition.

Payette nutrition screening scale

The payette nutrition screening scale (Fig. 3) (21) was developed from an in-depth study of nutritional-energy intake in elderly with declining functional status in the home setting. The scale is highly sensitive (78 %) and specific (77 %) in identifying individuals with intake deficits that could eventually result in weight loss or nutritional deficiency. The questionnaire is short, easily administered by healthcare professionals, and uses data on body mass, weight loss, pain as a cause of decreased functional status, vision, appetite, recent and stressful life events, and a list of the foods which are or are not eaten at breakfast. There are no laboratory investigations. The scores classify subjects into three categories of nutritional risk: high, intermediate, low. The scale screens for inadequate food intake but does not assess nutritional status. It was validated against 24 h dietary recall.

QUESTIONNAIRE TO ASSESS THE NEED FOR HELP WITH FOOD
IN THE ELDERLY

| Weight : | | lbs or | kg |
| Adult height : | ft | in or | m |

CIRCLE THE NUMBER CORRESPONDING TO THE STATEMENT THAT APPLIES TO THE CLIENT

THE CLIENT:

is very thin	Yes	2
	No	0
has lost weight in the last year	Yes	1
	No	0
suffers from arthritis to the point of interfering with daily activities	Yes	1
	No	0
has a quality of vision with glasses (if necessary) that is	Good	0
	Medium	1
	Poor	2
has a good appetite	Often	0
	Sometimes	1
	Never	2
recently suffered a stressful life event (e.g. personal illness / death of loved one)	Yes	1
	No	0

The client USUALLY consumes the foods below for breakfast

Fruit or fruit juice	Yes	0
	No	1
Eggs or cheese or peanut butter	Yes	0
	No	1
Bread or cereals	Yes	0
	No	1
Milk (1 cup or more than ¼ cup of coffee)	Yes	0
	No	1

TOTAL : _____

TOTAL SCORE		RECOMMENDATIONS
	Nutritional Risk	
6-13	High	Help with meal and snack preparation **AND** Referral to a dietician
3-5	Moderate	Regular monitoring of diet (checking on food intake, providing advice and encouragement)
0-2	Low	Regular monitoring for changes in risk factors (i.e., changed in health or weight loss)

Fig. 3. Payette nutrition screening scale (21).

Prognostic nutritional index

The prognostic nutritional index (PNI) (3) is a validated tool for assessing surgical inpatients for postoperative complication risk in terms of preoperative nutritional status using the following variables: tricipital skin thickness, serum albumin and transferrin, and a 4-antigen delayed cutaneous hypersensitivity test. The PNI expresses postoperative complication risk as a percentage: < 40 %: none; 40–49 %:

Sadness	Yesavage Geriatric Depression scale (≥ 15/30)
Cholesterol	< 4.14 mmol.l (160 mg/dl)
Albumin	< 40 g/L (4 g/dL)
Loss of weight	2 lb in 1 month or 5 lb in 6 months
Eat	eating problems (cognitive or physical)
Shopping	shopping problems or inability to prepare a meal

Fig. 4. Rapid office practice screen for risk of protein energy malnutrition (SCALES) (17).

moderate; ≥ 50 %: high. It can thus be used to select subjects requiring preoperative hyperalimentation in order to lower surgical complications.

Sadness-cholesterol-albumin-loss of weight-eat-shopping

The sadness–cholesterol–albumin–loss of weight–eat–shopping (SCALES) tool (Fig. 4) (17) is easily memorized by physicians, nurses or dieticians and quickly administered but requires laboratory data for cholesterol and albumin. It is a highly sensitive detector of malnutrition risk, and highlights the importance of depression in this regard. The SCALES correlates well with the MNA (19).

Subjective global assessment

The subjective global assessment (SGA) questionnaire (6, 7, 16) screens for weight loss and its direction (stable, ongoing, resolving), changes in eating behavior, gastrointestinal symptoms (anorexia, nausea, vomiting, and diarrhea), functional status, decrease in subcutaneous adipose tissue, muscle wasting, edema, and ascites. It results in a three-level classification: well-nourished, at risk of malnutrition, and poor nutritional status. The SGA is a sensitive and rapidly administered (2 min) tool for assessing nutritional complication risk in inpatients but precisely because it is subjective, the data are non-quantitative and, thus, cannot be used to monitor nutritional status.

Use of nutritional evaluation tools in clinical practice

Malnutrition screening in free-living elderly

Nutritional status should be monitored even in healthy elderly to detect and prevent deficits and their consequences. Primary prevention of this kind can be performed using the NSI, MNA, MNA-SF, NRS or NuRAS which identify those elderly at risk of malnutrition and give them the necessary information for improving their diet. The NuRAS and NRS are simple and rapid methods of identifying a number of malnutrition risk factors and providing medical and nutritional advice. The purpose of the NSI is awareness-raising rather than screening (28); also, as it is relatively nonspecific (27), it overestimates the number of persons at nutritional risk. The MNA is more discriminant: in the EURONUT SENECA study, the NSI identified 48 % of healthy elderly as being at high risk of malnutrition vs only 1 % using the MNA (12). Other studies using the MNA (29, 4) have confirmed that few free-living elderly are malnourished (0.5 %) but that the percentage increases (5.7 %) when they become institutionalized. Malnutrition may, therefore, be a predictive factor for institutionalization. The MNA-SF could be used as a screening tool for malnutrition risk by general practitioners in routine healthchecks of elderly persons. It could also be used as a marker of successful aging in the Rowe and Kahn classification (24). In the New Mexico study, MNA scores correlated with overall health status: very healthy elderly all scored > 24 (malnutrition risk threshold) (27.6 ± 1.82). Scores of 27–30 could be a marker of successful aging (31).

Malnutrition screening in frail or institutionalized elderly

The MNA can be used for nutritional assessment of frail or institutionalized elderly (26). Salva (29) showed that half the elderly in institutions are at risk of malnutrition. The MNA is highly sensitive (96 %) in evaluating nutritional status in frail elderly (8, 13). In frail free-living elderly, Payette's scale detects those requiring assistance with their dietary intake. In their study of 145 free-living elderly using home help services, Payette et al. found 24 % and 41 % at high or moderate risk of malnutrition, respectively (21).

Nutritional assessment in hospitalized elderly

MNA scores correlate with duration and cost of stay. A study in 166 inpatients > 70 years of age (24) showed that admission MNA scores < 17 correlated with hospital stays on average 10 days longer than those with MNA scores > 17. MNA scores also correlate with functional status during hospitalization, risk of bedsores, and transfer to an institution (5, 11, 23, 29). MNA nutritional status scores also correlate well with Mini Mental State scores, indicating that declining cognitive function can be responsible for declining nutritional status (11). The MNA is also useful for assessing nutritional status in nonhospitalized elderly such as those with Alzheimer's disease who are at particular risk: scores correlate with the weight loss often found in Alzheimer's disease (36). We have developed an education program which trains Alzheimer carers to monitor their relative's nutritional status using the MNA.

The PNI assesses complication risk in hospitalized elderly. Although useful in assessing operative risk and planning preoperative nutritional support (3, 32), it is long and expensive due to its reliance on hematological, biochemical, and immunological parameters. The SGA has also been recommended for assessing postoperative complication risk but is not elderly-specific; in addition, it requires training to administer and the ability to perform a clinical examination. The SCALES tool (17) assesses nutritional and functional status in hospitalized elderly and is highly sensitive but requires laboratory data such as plasma cholesterol and albumin; scores correlate well with the MNA.

Management and nutritional intervention guidelines using the MNA

The MNA was specifically designed to guide nutritional intervention by identifying the risk factors requiring correction.

- ▶ **MNA score ≥ 24** Satisfactory nutritional status. Reweigh 3-monthly. Offer basic balanced diet advice.
- ▶ **MNA score 17–23.5** Malnutrition risk with a good prognosis given early intervention. Analyze the MNA results to identify the reasons for the low score, i.e., examine those items where points are lost, e.g., if the patient is taking > 3 drugs daily (item 6), determine with their physician whether the number can be reduced. If the patient only takes two proper meals a day or is anorexic (items 11 and 14), determine whether they have an eating disorder. If the family cannot provide the meals, then arrange meals on wheels or domestic help. If the patient does not eat the requisite foods (fruits, vegetables, dairy products, meat) or take enough fluid (items 12–15), advise about varying the diet and offer domestic help and/or meals on wheels. For skin lesions (item 10), offer advice on high calorie and high protein supplements. Where possible, perform a detailed dietary interview. Follow up with a repeat MNA in 3 months.
- ▶ **MNA score < 17** Protein energy malnutrition. Analyze the score as described above. Perform a dietary interview. Investigate for other causes of malnutrition, e.g., depression, decreased functional status, or cognitive decline. Tailor advice to the MNA results and dietary interview: fractionate eating (more frequent meals and snacks, with less substance but greater nutritional density) and address the underlying causes. Repeat the MNA in 3 months.

We recently performed an MNA-assisted interventional study in retirement home elderly. Those scoring > 24 were not supplemented. Those scoring 17–23.5 were randomized into two groups with and without supplementation (300–500 kcal daily using varied high protein nutrient mixes). Those scoring < 17 were all supplemented. Supplementation was well accepted since approximately 400 kcal daily was ingested for 2 months. Most of the supplemented elderly increased their body weight and improved their MNA score at the end of the study. The study shows the utility of the MNA in nutritional assessment and follow-up (2).

Conclusion

Nutritional evaluation tools allow the early detection of malnutrition and should be integrated into the standard gerontological work-up (34). They help in planning preventive action and averting incipient malnutrition by rapid and appropriate nutritional intervention. In particular, the MNA not only assesses nutritional status but also guides nutritional intervention. It is, thus, the reference tool for diagnosing protein energy malnutrition in the elderly (18).

References

1. Alix E, Constans T (1998) Épidémiologie de la malnutrition protéino-énergétique (MPE) chez les personnes âgées. Année Gérontologique 12: 81–98
2. Arnaud-Battandier F, Lauque S, Paintin M (1998) MNA and nutritional intervention. In: Vellas B, Garry PJ, Guigoz Y (eds) Mini Nutritional Assessment (MNA): Research and Practice in Elderly. Nestlé Clinical and Performance Nutrition Workshop series, Vol 1, Lippincott-Raven, Philadelphia (in press)
3. Buzby GP, Mullen JL, Matthews DC, Hobbs CL, Rosato EF (1980) Prognostic nutritional index in gastrointestinal surgery. Am J Surg 139: 160–167
4. Chumlea C, Hall G, Lilly F, Siervogel RM, Guo S (1998) The Mini Nutritional Assessment and body composition in healthy adults. In: Vellas B, Garry PJ, Guigoz Y (eds) Mini Nutritional Assessment (MNA): Research and Practice in Elderly. Nestlé Clinical and Performance Nutrition Workshop series, Vol 1, Lippincott-Raven, Philadelphia (in press)
5. Cohendy R (1998) The Mini Nutritional Assessment for preoperative nutritional evaluation: a study on 419 elderly surgical patients. In: Vellas B, Garry PJ, Guigoz Y (eds) Mini Nutritional Assessment (MNA): Research and Practice in Elderly. Nestlé Clinical and Performance Nutrition Workshop series, Vol 1, Lippincott-Raven, Philadelphia (in press)
6. Detsky AS, McLaughlin JR, Baker JP, Johnston N, Whittaker S, Mendelson RA, Jeejeebhoy KN (1987) What is subjective assessment of nutritional status? J Parent Enteral Nutr 11: 8–13
7. Detsky AS, Smalley PS, Chang J (1994) Is this patient malnourished? JAMA 271: 54–58
8. Donini LM, De Felice MR, Deon F (1998) MNA in a population of a frail elderly. In: Vellas B, Garry PJ, Guigoz Y (eds) Mini Nutritional Assessment (MNA): Research and Practice in Elderly. Nestlé Clinical and performance Nutrition Workshop series, Vol 1, Lippincott-Raven, Philadelphia (in press)
9. Dwyer J (1994) Strategies to detect and prevent malnutrition in the elderly: the Nutrition Screening Initiative. Nutrition Today 5: 14–24
10. Gazzotti C, Pepinster A, Petermans J, Albert A (1997) Interobserver agreement on MNA nutritional scale of hospitalized elderly patients. J Nutr Health Aging 1: 23–27
11. Gazotti C, Pepinster A, Petermans J (1998) Diagnostic and prognostic efficiency of MNA nutritional scale in geriatric hospitalized patients. In: Vellas B, Garry PJ, Guigoz Y (eds) Mini Nutritional Assessment (MNA): Research and Practice in Elderly. Nestlé Clinical and Performance Nutrition Workshop series, Vol 1, Lippincott-Raven, Philadelphia (in press)
12. Groot CPGM, Lier AV, Prompers J, Van Staveren WA (1998) Evaluating the NSI and MNA as tools for assessing the nutritional situation of elderly people. In: Vellas B, Garry PJ, Guigoz Y (eds) Mini Nutritional Assessment (MNA): Research and Practice in Elderly. Nestlé Clinical and Performance Nutrition Workshop series, Vol 1, Lippincott-Raven, Philadelphia (in press)
13. Guigoz Y, Vellas B (1995) Test d'évaluation de l'état nutritionnel de la personne âgée: le Mini Nutritional Assessment. Med Hyg 53: 1965–1969
14. Guigoz Y, Vellas B, Garry PJ (1997) Mini Nutritional Assessment: a practical assessment tool for grading the nutritional state of elderly patients. Facts, Research and Intervention in Geriatrics [suppl Nutrition in the Elderly, 3rd ed: The Mini Nutritional Assessment (MNA), Vellas BJ, Guigoz Y, Garry PJ, Albarède JL eds]: pp. 15–60
15. Hickson M, Hill M (1997) Implementing a nutritional assessment tool in the community: a report describing the process, audit and problems encountered. J Hum Nut Diet 10: 373–377
16. Ireton-Jones CS, Hase JM (1992) Comprehensive nutritional assessment: the dietitian's contribution to the team effort. Nutrition 2: 75–81

17. Morley JE (1993) Why do physicians fail to recognize and treat malnutrition in older persons? J Am Geriatr Soc 39: 1139–1140
18. Morley JE (1997) Anorexia of aging: physiologic and pathologic. Am J Clin Nutr 66: 760–773
19. Morley JE, Miller DK, Perry HM, Guigoz Y, Vellas B (1997) Anorexia of aging, leptin and the Mini Nutritional Assessment. In: Vellas B, Garry PJ, Guigoz Y (eds) Mini Nutritional Assessment (MNA): Research and Practice in Elderly. Nestlé Clinical and Performance Nutrition Workshop series, Vol 1, Lippincott-Raven, Philadelphia (in press)
20. Nikolaus T, Bach M, Siezen S, Volhert D, Oster P, Schlierf G (1995) Assessment of nutritional risk in the elderly. Ann Nutr Metab 39: 340–345
21. Payette H, Gray-Donald K, Cyr R, Coulombe C, Boutier V (1996) Efficacy of a nutritional screening tool in free-living frail elderly. Age Nutr 7: 168
22. Prendergast JM, Coe RM, Chavez MN, Romeis JC, Miller DK, Wolinsky FD (1989) Clinical validation of a nutritional risk index. J Community Health 3: 125–135
23. Quadri P, Fraggiacomo C, Pertoldi W, Guigoz Y, Herrmann F, Rapin CH (1998) MNA and cost of care. In: Vellas B, Garry PJ, Guigoz Y (eds) Mini Nutritional Assessment (MNA): Research and Practice in Elderly. Nestlé Clinical and performance Nutrition Workshop series, Vol 1, Lippincott-Raven, Philadelphia (in press)
24. Rowe JW, Kahn RL (1997) Successful aging. Gerontologist 37: 433–440
25. Rubenstein LZ (1998) Development of a short version of the Mini Nutritional Assessment. In: Vellas B, Garry PJ, Guigoz Y (eds) Mini Nutritional Assessment (MNA): Research and Practice in Elderly. Nestlé Clinical and performance Nutrition Workshop series, Vol 1, Lippincott-Raven, Philadelphia (in press)
26. Rudman D, Feller AG (1989) Protein-calorie undernutrition in the nursing home. J Am Geriatr Soc 37: 173–183
27. Rush D (1997) Nutrition screening in old people: its place in a coherent practice of preventive health care. Annu Rev Nutr 17: 101–125
28. Sahyoun NR, Jacques PF, Dallal GE, Russell RM (1997) Nutrition Screening Initiative Checklist may be a better awareness/educational tool than a screening one. J Am Diet Assoc 97: 760–764
29. Salva A, Bleda J, Bolibar I, Perez M (1998) The Mini Nutritional Assessment in clinical practice. In: Vellas B, Garry PJ, Guigoz Y (eds) Mini Nutritional Assessment (MNA): Research and Practice in Elderly. Nestlé Clinical and performance Nutrition Workshop series, Vol 1, Lippincott-Raven, Philadelphia (in press)
30. Sheirlinkx K, Rolland Y, Nourhashemi F (1998) Les différents programmes d'évaluation gérontologiques: revue de la littérature. Evaluation Gérontologique (Collection L'Année Gérontologique), Serdi, Paris (in press)
31. Sheirlinkx K, Nicolas AS, Nourhashemi F, Vellas B, Albarède JL, Garry P (1998) The MNA score in successfully aging persons. In: Vellas B, Garry PJ, Guigoz Y (eds) Mini Nutritional Assessment (MNA): Research and Practice in Elderly. Nestlé Clinical and performance Nutrition Workshop series, Vol 1, Lippincott-Raven, Philadelphia (in press)
32. Smith RC, Hartemink R (1988) Improvement of nutritional measures during preoperative parenteral nutrition in patients selected by the prognostic nutritional index: a randomized controlled trial. J Parent Enteral Nutr 12: 587–591
33. Stuck AE, Siu AL, Wieland GD, Adams J, Rubenstein LZ (1993) Comprehensive geriatric assessment: a meta-analysis of controlled trials. Lancet 342: 1032–1036
34. Vellas B, Albarède JL (1997) Nutritional assessment as part of the geriatric evaluation: The Mini Nutritional Assessment. Facts, Research and Intervention in Geriatrics [suppl Nutrition in the Elderly, 3rd ed: The Mini Nutritional Assessment (MNA), Vellas BJ, Guigoz Y, Garry PJ, Albarède JL eds]: pp 11–13
35. White JV, Dwyer JT, Posner BM, Ham RJ, Lipschitz DA, Wellman NS (1992) Nutrition Screening Initiative: development and implementation of the public awareness checklist and screening tools. J Am Diet Assoc 92: 163–167

36. White H, Pieper C, Shmader K, Fillenbaum G (1996) Weight change in Alzheimer disease. J Am Geriatr Soc 44: 265–272
37. Wolinsky FD, Coe RM, McIntosh WA, Kubena KS, Prendergast JM, Chavez MN, Miller DK, Romeis JC, Landmann WA (1990) Progress in the development of a nutritional risk index. J Nutr 120: 1549–1553

Author's address:

Monsieur le Professeur Vellas
Service de Médecine Interne et de Gérontologie Clinique
170 avenue de Casselardit
31300 Toulouse, France

Diagnosis of zinc deficiency*

H.-P. Roth, M. Kirchgessner

Institute for Nutritional Physiology, Technical University, Munich, Germany

Summary

Though far more common, particularly in elderly people, than was previously assumed, marginal zinc deficiency does not lead to the classical manifestations of zinc deficiency and is therefore difficult to diagnose. There is therefore a need for sensitive parameters that can reliably demonstrate even marginal zinc deficiency, as suboptimal zinc status can seriously impair human health, performance, reproductive functions, and mental and physical development. The most important criteria for the diagnosis of zinc deficiency are critically discussed. The laboratory parameters currently considered to be the most useful indicators of marginal zinc deficiency are zinc-binding capacity and serum/plasma alkaline phosphatase activity before and after zinc supplementation (zinc tolerance test!). In order to obtain a reliable assessment of a patients zinc status, a number of different diagnostic parameters should always be measured.

Introduction

Zinc is an essential trace element that has a variety of biochemical functions in enzymes and other proteins, nucleic acids, hormones, and the immune system. Dietary deficiency of it therefore interferes with many metabolic processes. Nevertheless, manifest dietary deficiency of zinc in humans, as was seen in the 1960s in Egypt and in the 1970s in Iran, occurs only rarely and under extreme circumstances. In the industrialized countries of Europe and in the USA, adequate dietary intake of zinc makes the occurrence of any significant manifestations of zinc deficiency (Table 1) unlikely. Nevertheless, epidemiological studies in the USA and Germany have shown that latent forms of zinc deficiency are considerably more common than was previously assumed. For example, the zinc intake of adults in Germany was shown to have fallen by 20–25 % over a period of eight years (1988–1996), indicating that zinc intake in Germany can be marginal and should be increased (28).

---

* This contribution was translated from German to English by David Playfair, 30 Cheverton Road, London N19 3AY, Great Britain, Email: DavidPlayfair@compuserve.com

Table 1. Manifestations of zinc deficiency in humans and animals

	Animals	Humans
Growth retardation	+	+
Delayed or absent sexual maturation	+	+
Zinc deficiency during pregnancy		
Abortions	+	–
Malformations	+	–
Disturbed maternal behaviour	+	–
Anorexia	+	+
Diarrhoea	+	+
Impaired immune system	+	(–)
Increased susceptibility to infections	+	+
Delayed wound healing	+	(+)
Parakeratosis	+	+
Bone changes	+	(–)
Hair loss	+	+
Reduced sense of taste and smell	+	+
Impaired learning behaviour, irritability, aggressivity	+	(–)
Mental lethargy	+	(–)

+ proven; – not adequately investigated; (+) probable; (–) conjectured

Table 2. Possible causes of dietary zinc deficiency

1) Inadequate dietary supply due to
   a) poor or deficient diet (high sugar consumption, white bread, etc.)
   b) unbalanced reduction diets (low zinc intake, catabolism)
   c) alcoholism
   d) parenteral nutrition

2) Reduced zinc absorption due to
   a) reduced bioavailability of dietary zinc due to dietary factors (phytin-rich vegetarian food, high raw fibre content)
   b) increased intake of calcium or polyphosphates
   c) genetically determined disturbances of absorption (acrodermatitis enteropathica, Crohn's disease, coeliac disease)
   d) renal diseases (absent tubular resorption)

3) Increased zinc requirement due to
   a) pregnancy (uptake of zinc by foetus)
   b) lactation (increased zinc loss)
   c) rapid growth in children and adolescents (increased zinc deposition)
   d) physical exertion (e.g. competitive sport)

4) Increased zinc elimination due to
   a) diabetes mellitus, sickle cell anaemia (increased renal elimination of zinc)
   b) hepatic and renal diseases (increased renal elimination of zinc)
   c) diarrhoea (increased faecal elimination of zinc)
   d) burns, inflammation , dialysis (exudation, catabolism)
   e) operations, surgical procedures (blood loss, catabolism)
   f) infections, parasitic ulceration (chronic blood loss)
   g) corticosteroid therapy, oral contraceptives (increased renal elimination of zinc)
   h) chelating agents, diuretics (increased renal elimination of zinc)
   i) increased sweat loss (competitive sport)

Causes of zinc deficiency

The fact that zinc intake in Germany is falling may be largely due to increased consumption of industrially processed and therefore zinc-poor foods such as white sugar, polished rice, and finely milled flour and to changes in dietary habits such as reduced meat consumption. A typical modern diet that could lead to zinc deficiency might thus consist of white bread, fat, and Cola. Partial replacement of animal protein with vegetable protein also reduces the absorption and thus body levels of zinc. Nevertheless, marginal zinc deficiency that does not give rise to any clinical manifestations is difficult to diagnose even though it can impair human and animal health, performance, reproductive functions, and mental and physical development. The extent to which the body's zinc requirement is met by the diet depends not just on the amount of zinc ingested, but also largely on the extent to which ingested zinc is absorbed. Zinc deficiency can also result from increased requirement, reduced utilization, or increased loss, as may occur in certain genetically determined diseases. As seen from Table 2, the possible causes of zinc deficiency are many and varied.

Children, adolescents, pregnant and lactating women, competitive sportsmen and women, vegetarians, alcoholics, the elderly, people who are ill, patients who have recently undergone surgery, and convalescing patients should therefore be regarded as high-risk groups for zinc deficiency. For a variety of reasons, zinc deficiency is especially liable to occur in the elderly. The zinc requirement of older people may not be met because of difficulties in chewing and swallowing, physical and mental impairments, medications, frequent illness, poor appetite, and changes in the absorption, metabolism, and elimination of zinc. These various factors can lead to deficits in zinc metabolism such as a reduction in the zinc content of leucocytes. This in turn may partially explain the increased susceptibility of older people to infections. Similarly, some of the skin changes commonly found in geriatric patients are typical manifestations of dietary zinc deficiency. The use of zinc-containing preparations is therefore becoming increasingly common particularly in geriatric patients, as it may exert a positive influence on aging phenomena. Thus, administration of zinc has been shown to improve the function of the immune system and to reduce the severity and duration of influenza and colds. Zinc administration has also been shown to improve other symptoms of illness and functional disorders such as taste disturbances, impaired wound healing, skin diseases, and hair loss. Early disturbance of glucose utilization (diabetes mellitus type II) and psychiatric disorders including depression in geriatric patients have also been considerably improved by zinc supplementation. Zinc supplementation is also useful in rheumatism and all inflammatory and chronic diseases, in particular those of the gastrointestinal tract and liver, and in alcohol abuse. The diagnosis of latent zinc deficiency therefore calls for the use of sensitive parameters that indicate even small deviations from physiological requirements. Zinc deficiency is understood to mean a reduction in total body zinc to below the normal level, leading to abnormal physiological and biochemical functions that can be corrected by zinc supplementation.

Table 3. Possible criteria for the diagnosis of zinc deficiency

1) Zinc level in tissues
  a) Bone
  b) Hair
  c) Zinc balance studies
	4) ^{65}Zn uptake by erythrocytes
	5) Activity of zinc metalloenzymes
	6) Protein concentrations
	  a) Metallothionein

2) Zinc level in body fluids
  a) Plasma
  b) Urine
  c) Saliva
	b) Thymulin
	  c) Insulin, IGF-1
	  d) Zinc-binding capacity
	7) Response to zinc supplementation

3) Zinc level in blood elements
  a) Erythrocytes
  b) Platelets
  c) Leucocytes
	a) Serum zinc
	  b) Serum activity of alkaline phosphatase
	  c) Zinc-binding capacity
	  d) ^{65}Zn uptake by erythrocytes

Assessment of zinc status

The zinc status of human beings is difficult to determine because of the absence to date of any suitable marker that reacts both specifically and sensitively even to marginal changes in zinc intake and zinc content of the body. Table 3 shows the parameters that have been used to date to assess the zinc status of humans and animals. The use of animal models for the induction of genuine dietary zinc deficiency is very important, as only in this way can the usefulness of a method or parameter be tested. The various groups of parameters that can be used as indices of zinc status are discussed below.

Zinc level in tissues

The introduction of flame and graphite-furnace atomic absorption spectroscopy has provided a rapid and sensitive method for the routine determination of zinc. The zinc status of an individual can be assessed either by determination of total body zinc or indirectly by determination of the zinc content of a suitable body compartment. Muscle (60 %) and bone (30 %) are the most important compartments for zinc, between them accounting for almost 90 % of total body zinc. Zinc deficiency has little influence on the zinc concentration of soft tissues, as shown by the fact that the zinc concentration of the muscle of laboratory rats was shown to remain constant despite severe experimental zinc deficiency. By contrast, the zinc concentration of bone falls by up to 70 % in the presence of experimental zinc deficiency (29). Determination of the zinc content of bone under standardized experimental conditions is therefore regarded as the method of choice for assessing the zinc status of animals (20, 36, 37). Unfortunately, the need to take bone biopsies excludes the use of this method for routine determinations in humans.

In a number of studies the zinc content of hair has been used as an indicator of the zinc status of the individual. Unfortunately, although hair has the advantage of being an easily accessible tissue, it is of no diagnostic value in relation to zinc deficiency. To date no serious study has provided any scientific evidence to support the use of zinc analysis of hair for this purpose (15). This is not only because there is great intra- and interindividual variation in hair growth periods, but also because the zinc content of hair can be influenced by a variety of exogenous factors such as shampoos, hair dyes, hair bleaches, hair strengtheners, toiletry products, cosmetics, and a host of environmental factors. Other influences include geographical location, race, time of year, age, growth rate, state of health, medications, breast-feeding, etc. As a result of all these influencing variables, the zinc content of hair is of no diagnostic value in relation to the zinc status of an individual. Nor has the zinc content of fingernails proved to be any more useful as an indicator of an individuals zinc status. By contrast, the zinc balance of an animal or human is a very accurate reflection of zinc status, a negative balance indicating low zinc status and a positive balance indicating an adequate dietary intake of zinc. Unfortunately, determination of the zinc balance of humans is time-consuming and technically difficult and is therefore not suitable for general clinical use.

Zinc level in plasma or serum

Because it is so easily accessible, plasma or serum is the body fluid most commonly used as a biopsy material for determination of zinc status. Nevertheless, the use of plasma or serum zinc level as an indicator of zinc status is complicated by the fact that as a result of homeostatic regulation, bodily zinc is mobilized when supply is inadequate and plasma zinc therefore changes only when this homeostatic capacity has been exhausted (14). Some authors therefore feel that plasma or serum zinc level is not a good parameter for assessing zinc status, especially as circulating zinc accounts for less than 1 % of total body zinc (45). Furthermore, plasma zinc can vary independently of zinc status in a large number of pathological conditions including stress, infections, myocardial infarction, physical exertion, and pregnancy, and also in association with changes in hormone status. As the amount of information available on individual patients is often limited, it is therefore often very difficult to know whether a low plasma level of zinc is due to genuine zinc deficiency. Under carefully controlled experimental conditions the plasma or serum level of zinc is of course a useful indicator of the individual zinc status of a person or animal (25, 32). Despite the fact that serum zinc concentration is known to be inadequate as an indicator of zinc status (45), serum continues to be the material most frequently used for the assessment of zinc status. The zinc concentration of whole blood should not be used as an indicator of zinc status, as in rats with severe zinc deficiency 85 % of the zinc loss from whole blood was found to be due to zinc loss from serum (35). Although renal elimination of zinc is reduced in zinc deficiency, determination of the zinc content of a 24-hour urine specimen can be no more than an aid to the diagnosis of zinc deficiency, and even then only if conditions such as cirrhosis of the liver, sickle cell anaemia, chronic renal diseases, and other causes of hyperzincuria can be excluded. Similarly, the zinc concentration of saliva was found not to be a sensitive indicator of zinc intake in pregnant women and women with low zinc status.

Zinc level in blood elements

Erythrocytes

Another parameter that has been suggested for use as an indicator of zinc status is the zinc content of blood cells. In adult humans the proportion of total body zinc located in the blood is less than 0.5 %. Of this, 12–22 % is in the plasma, 75–88 % in erythrocytes, and about 3 % in leucocytes and platelets. The available reports on the zinc concentration of blood cells in patients with zinc deficiency are highly contradictory. As the mean lifespan of erythrocytes is around 120 days, the zinc level of erythrocytes does not reflect short-term changes in zinc status and therefore can function at best only as a long-term indicator. In studies on humans (19, 27, 40), controlled zinc depletion by consumption of low-zinc diets over periods of four to eight weeks led to no changes in the zinc content of erythrocytes. In studies on rats, even severe experimental zinc deficiency over periods of several weeks likewise failed to lead to any reduction in erythrocyte zinc content (2, 3, 17).

Platelets

Use of platelets as a tool for assessing zinc status was proposed by Pai & Prasad (23). As platelets have a shorter half-life (around 18 days) than erythrocytes, platelet zinc level might potentially be useful as an indicator of acute changes in zinc status. However, the few studies that have been performed on this question have failed to demonstrate any change in platelet zinc levels after experimental zinc depletion either in humans (19, 40) or in animals (18, 41).

Leucocytes

In theory, leucocyte zinc levels might likewise be a useful indicator of zinc status. However, leucocytes consist of a number of subgroups of different morphology, function, lifespan, and zinc content. For example, the half-life of neutrophils is six to seven hours, whereas that of monocytes is one to three days, and the zinc content of monocytes is higher than that of polymorphs. The zinc content of a pure cell population should therefore be a more reliable indicator of zinc status than that of the leucocyte population as a whole. Nevertheless, it is very doubtful whether the zinc content of leucocytes or even of specific types of leucocytes is a better indicator of zinc status than is serum zinc level. In any case, separation of the various subpopulations of leucocytes and determination of their zinc content is technically complex and time consuming. The zinc concentration of blood cells such as granulocytes, lymphocytes, and monocytes is low (21) and the risk of contamination with exogenous zinc is very high. In addition, care must be taken to ensure that no clumping of cells occurs, as with electronic cell counting and expression of results as nanograms of zinc per 10^6 cells this would result in overestimation of zinc content. Even after washing, the monocyte fraction is often contaminated with zinc-rich platelets, and estimates of monocyte zinc level can be correspondingly false. Use of the zinc levels of individual blood cell fractions as indicators of zinc status is further complicated by the changes in zinc content that occur in haematological diseases and the variations in the relative proportions of the various subclasses of cells that occur during pregnancy and in various pathological states such as burns, inflammation, and infections. In studies on zinc-deficient animals, leucocyte zinc levels were not found to be reduced (1, 5, 17). In patients with various conditions known to lead to marginal zinc status, such as cirrhosis, cancer, and endocrine and rheumatic diseases, the zinc concentrations of the mononuclear and polymorphonuclear cell fractions of leucocytes were found to be no more sensitive or reliable than plasma zinc as indicators of zinc status (24). In a controlled seven-week zinc depletion and repletion study on young men (40), the zinc concentrations of neutrophils, platelets, and erythrocytes showed no reaction to changes in zinc status even though the onset of marginal zinc deficiency was demonstrated via reduced zinc concentration in the plasma (39). Even in hospitalized elderly patients whose plasma zinc concentrations were significantly lower than those of younger control patients, no differences were found in terms of the zinc content of mononuclear or polymorphonuclear leucocytes (8). In many clinical situations this expensive and time-consuming method is therefore not useful for identifying marginal zinc deficiency, especially as to our knowledge a reduction in the zinc content of the blood cells of zinc-deficient animals has never been demonstrated under standardized and controlled experimental conditions despite repeated attempts to do so (17).

^{65}Zn uptake by blood cells

Another possible method for assessing zinc status is determination of the in vitro uptake of zinc by blood cells under standard physiological conditions. The in vitro uptake of zinc by whole blood, erythrocytes, and leucocytes has been found to be inversely proportional to dietary zinc intake and plasma zinc concentration, i.e. to be highest when plasma zinc concentration is lowest. The ^{65}Zn uptake of blood cells is simpler to determine than are low concentrations of zinc in blood cells. An in vitro test has the additional advantage that it does not expose the patient to any radioactivity.

Increased in vitro uptake of ^{65}Zn by erythrocytes was found to be a sensitive and specific indicator of zinc deficiency in the rat model (31, 46). After administration of a zinc-deficient diet to rats for 26 days the zinc concentration of platelets was unchanged, whereas the in vivo uptake of ^{65}Zn by the platelets of the zinc-deficient rats after a zinc injection had increased by a factor of three (41). In another study, the in vitro uptake of ^{65}Zn by erythrocytes under standard conditions in a physiological medium was found to be a suitable method for identifying early subclinical zinc deficiency (22, 46).

Activity of zinc metalloenzymes

Changes in the activity of zinc-dependent enzymes have been used as a biochemical indicator of the zinc status of humans and animals. However, studies on rats have shown that only some of the known zinc metalloenzymes, e.g. serum alkaline phosphatase and blood carbonic anhydrase, are sensitive to a zinc-deficient diet, whereas others retain full activity even in the presence of extreme zinc deficiency (12, 13).

A large number of studies have now demonstrated a relationship between serum alkaline phosphatase activity and dietary zinc intake. Along with serum zinc, this parameter has therefore become the most commonly used biochemical indicator of zinc status in humans and animals. Determination of serum or plasma alkaline phosphatase activity has proved to be a useful, easily performed, and high-through-put screening test for low zinc status (30, 32). Unfortunately, serum alkaline phosphatase activity, like zinc concentration in serum or blood cells, can be influenced by a variety of factors such as liver function, bone turnover, and calcium status; hence it is difficult to establish normal values. The response of serum alkaline phosphatase activity to zinc supplementation (see response to zinc supplementation below) is therefore a more useful parameter for detecting marginal zinc deficiency in humans.

Protein concentrations

Although the biological function of metallothionein is not yet precisely understood, it has been suggested that metallothionein, a low molecular weight zinc-binding protein with a high cysteine content (30 %) and a metal-binding capacity of 7 gram-atoms of zinc per mole, might be a reliable indicator of zinc status. The metallothionein concentration of tissues is often proportional to zinc status, falling to below the limit of detection during zinc depletion and rising again after zinc repletion. In a study on adult men, the metallothionein concentration of erythrocytes fell by 46 % during zinc depletion and rose again during repletion (44). In a study on young men, supplementation with 50 mg zinc per day led after only eight days to a significant rise in the metallothionein concentration of erythrocytes as compared with that in a control group (42). Although precise and reliable assay of metallothionein levels in tissues and biological fluids is very promising as a means of assessing an individual's zinc status, further studies are required in order to determine what variables influence this assay, as only on the basis of this knowledge can the potential of metallothionein for the detection of zinc deficiency in humans be properly assessed.

The serum level of the thymic hormone thymulin has also been proposed as a possible indicator of early zinc deficiency in humans. In a study on men, experimental zinc deficiency led to a significant fall in serum thymulin activity, while subsequent zinc supplementation led to normalization of levels both in vivo and in vitro (26). Determination of thymulin activity was found to be a sensitive indicator of zinc status in undernourished children with marginal zinc deficiency (10). Further studies are required in order to determine whether the fall in thymulin level that occurs in experimental zinc deficiency (7) can really be exploited to develop a simple method for assessing zinc deficiency in humans. The same applies to the reduced serum levels of insulin and insulin-like growth factor-1 (IGF-1) found in rats with experimentally induced zinc deficiency (36, 37).

The zinc present in serum/plasma is distributed between two principal fractions, namely zinc bound strongly to α_2-macroglobulin (1/3) and that bound weakly to albumin (2/3). The rapid initial fall in plasma zinc that follows dietary zinc restriction is probably due to separation of the weakly bound fraction from albumin, whereas the strongly-bound fraction remains bound even in extreme zinc deficiency (38). The relative number of free zinc-binding sites on albumin could therefore function as an indicator of the zinc status of a human or animal. Under experimental conditions the percentage zinc-binding capacity of the serum of rats was found to be a good indicator of dietary zinc intake (33).

Response to zinc supplementation

Serum/plasma zinc level and alkaline phosphatase activity are currently the most commonly employed indicators of zinc status. However, as stated above, under practical conditions these parameters are subject to a variety of influences; hence it is difficult to establish normal values for them. This problem can nevertheless be circumvented by using techniques that measure response. The most sensitive laboratory criteria currently used for diagnosing zinc deficiency in humans and animals are therefore defined clinical or biochemical reactions to zinc supplementation under controlled conditions (9, 31–34).

As a result of homeostatic regulation of plasma zinc concentration, a low zinc intake leads firstly to increased absorption and then to reduced excretion of zinc (14, 43, 47). This is achieved by a variety of zinc transporters (16) and intracellular binding proteins that regulate both the absorption and the cellular influx and efflux of zinc (42). These adaptive mechanisms maintain normal plasma levels of zinc over a broad range of zinc intake levels (14). Supplementation with physiological amounts of zinc will barely alter the plasma zinc concentration of an individual whose zinc intake is already adequate (32). On the other hand, excessive doses of zinc can cause plasma zinc concentration to rise briefly, even in individuals without zinc deficiency, until the regulatory mechanisms exert their full effect. The zinc tolerance test, i.e. detection of an unequivocal rise in serum zinc after oral administration of zinc, has therefore proved to be a very good indicator of zinc status in both young and geriatric patients of both sexes (4).

Current zinc status is most closely mirrored by the serum level of alkaline phosphatase (EC 3.1.3.1), a zinc metalloenzyme whose activity falls rapidly and profoundly in the presence of zinc deficiency and rises back towards a plateau when adequate zinc intake is restored (32). Where oral administration or – as in the studies referred to here (32, 34) – injections of zinc lead to an increase in serum alkaline phosphatase activity, then, depending on the size of the increase recorded, a greater or lesser degree of zinc deficiency must have been present, as in individuals whose zinc status is adequate administration of additional zinc does not lead to an increase in the activity of this enzyme (Table 4). In studies on rats in which precisely defined degrees of zinc deficiency had been induced by controlling dietary zinc intake (32, 34), it was shown that using this response technique it is possible to diagnose not just zinc deficiency, but also suboptimal zinc status, i.e. a degree of inadequacy of zinc supply that is by its nature very difficult to diagnose. In a study on patients with manifestations of zinc deficiency following prolonged total parenteral nutrition, the response of alkaline phosphatase to zinc supplementation was found to be a useful indicator of subclinical zinc deficiency (11).

Table 4. Serum alkaline phosphatase activity in rats with different dietary zinc intakes before and three days after an intraperitoneal injection of zinc[1] (32)

Zinc content of diet (mg Zn/kg DM)	Alkaline phosphatase activity (mU/ml)		Percentage rise (%)
	28th day of study (before Zn injection)	31st day of study (after Zn injection)	
1.3	23 ± 8	152 ± 36	560
4	39 ± 10	162 ± 35	315
6	88 ± 41	195 ± 61	122
8	116 ± 19	185 ± 72	59
10	139 ± 29	193 ± 33	39
12	183 ± 44	245 ± 62	34
20	175 ± 39	249 ± 66	42
100	239 ± 27	246 ± 50	3

[1] 0.8 mg Zn/animal; n = 112

As stated in the section Protein concentrations above, under experimental conditions the percentage zinc-binding capacity of serum was found to be a good indicator of deficient dietary intake of zinc (33). In this in vitro test the percentage zinc-binding capacity of serum was found to be inversely proportional to dietary and serum levels of zinc (Table 5). The relative number of free zinc-binding sites on serum/plasma albumin and transferrin is therefore used as an indicator of zinc status. Percentage zinc-binding capacity is preferable to serum zinc level for the assessment of zinc status, as when zinc supply is adequate percentage zinc-binding capacity reaches a constant level of 60–70 % and does not rise further in response to additional doses of zinc. Because percentage zinc-binding capacity remains constant, this in vitro method of assessing the zinc status of animals or humans does not require zinc supplementation. In a study on insulin-dependent diabetics who had developed zinc deficiency as a result of excessive renal excretion of zinc, zinc supplementation led to normalization of the zinc-binding capacity of plasma

Table 5. Percentage zinc-binding capacity and serum zinc level in rats on different dietary zinc intakes before and after an injection of zinc[1] (33)

Zn content of diet (mg Zn/kg DM)	Before zinc injection		After zinc injection	
	Zinc-binding capacity (%)	Serum Zn level (µg Zn/ml)	Zinc-binding capacity (%)	Serum Zn level (µg Zn/ml)
1.3	87.1 ± 2.7	0.40 ± 0.09	70.4 ± 2.0	0.93 ± 0.03
4	89.1 ± 3.5	0.40 ± 0.16	76.6 ± 2.3	0.76 ± 0.08
6	84.3 ± 2.1	0.42 ± 0.14	71.4 ± 3.8	0.78 ± 0.12
8	83.8 ± 1.1	0.43 ± 0.02	74.0 ± 3.5	0.71 ± 0.13
10	74.2 ± 4.8	0.61 ± 0.11	67.4 ± 3.1	1.13 ± 0.15
12	74.8 ± 3.1	0.63 ± 0.10	69.8 ± 2.4	0.95 ± 0.06
20	69.2 ± 3.7	0.84 ± 0.08	70.0 ± 3.3	0.97 ± 0.17
100	58.9 ± 5.3	1.26 ± 0.10	61.2 ± 3.8	1.24 ± 0.08

[1] 0.8 mg Zn/animal; n = 112

(6). In this study the zinc-binding capacity of plasma was found to be more sensitive than plasma zinc level as an indicator of zinc status.

In vitro uptake of ^{65}Zn by erythrocytes after zinc supplementation is another possible method for diagnosing inadequate dietary zinc intake (31); however it is time-consuming, assumes the existence of an isotope laboratory, and provides no additional information as compared with alkaline phosphatase activity or the percentage zinc-binding capacity of serum.

Conclusions

Many of the parameters described here have been found in standardized animal experiments to be sensitive indicators of marginal zinc status. Under practical conditions, however, they are often of only limited usefulness for the assessment of zinc status in humans. This is because in most cases either the individual's precise dietary and medical history – and thus many important factors that influence zinc status – are unknown, or the tests are too complex and expensive to perform on a routine basis, or acquisition of the necessary biological samples is impracticable in humans. As the laboratory tests described here can be influenced in different ways by a wide variety of diseases, the best advice that can be given at present is not to rely exclusively on any one indicator, but rather to use a number of indicators in order to derive more reliable conclusions as to an individual's zinc status. At present the best indicators of possible dietary zinc deficiency are serum/plasma alkaline phosphatase activity and, with reservations, serum zinc concentration after zinc supplementation and serum zinc-binding capacity. For human zinc supplementation we use well-tolerated organic zinc compounds such as D-gluconate, DL-aspartate, histidinate, and orotate rather than the inorganic salt zinc sulphate. In order to induce a reliable and specific response of the proposed parameters for the purpose of assessing zinc status in humans, supplementation with 20–25 mg zinc twice daily one to two hours before a meal for four days is recommended. On the fifth day, 24 hours after the last dose of zinc, the various diagnostic parameters should be determined and compared with the corresponding values before zinc supplementation. Where zinc status is found to be marginal, supplementation with 20–25 mg zinc per day for three months is recommended, after which period the various parameters should be checked to see whether they have returned to normal. Nevertheless, there remains a pressing need for a simple, clinically practicable method that can rapidly and reliably determine the zinc status of an individual and indicate impending zinc deficiency.

References

1. Apgar J, Fitzgerald JA (1987) Measure of zinc status in ewes given a low zinc diet throughout pregnancy. Nutr Res 7: 1281–1290
2. Bettger WJ, Taylor CG (1986) Effects of copper and zinc status of rats on the concentration of copper and zinc in the erythrocyte membrane. Nutr Res 6: 451–457
3. Boge E, Roth H-P, Kirchgessner M (1992) Zur Verteilung des Zinks im Blut von an Zink depletierten Ratten. J Anim Physiol a Anim Nutr 67: 225–229

4. Capel ID, Spencer EP, Daivies AE, Levitt HN (1982) The assessment of zinc status by the zinc tolerance test in various groups of patients. Clin Biochem 15: 257–260
5. Crofton RW, Clapham M, Humphries WR, Aggett PJ, Mills CF (1983) Leucocyte and tissue zinc concentration in the growing pig. Proc Nutr Soc 42: 128A
6. Cunningham JJ, Fu A, Mearkle PL, Brown RG (1994) Hyperzincuria in individuals with insulin-dependent diabetes mellitus: current zinc status and the effect of high-dose zinc supplementation. Metabolism 43: 1558–1562
7. Dardenne M, Wade S, Savino W, Nabarra B, Prasad AS, Bach J-F (1988) Thymulin and zinc deficiency. In: Essential and Toxic Trace Elements in Human Health and Disease. Prasad AS, ed. Alan R Liss, New York 329–336
8. Goode HF, Kelleher J, Walker BE (1990) A critical assessment of leucocyte zinc as an index of Zn status in chronically ill hospitalized elderly patients. Proc Nutr Soc 49: 71A
9. Halsted JA, Smith JC, Irwin MI (1974) A conspectus of research on zinc requirements of man. J Nutr 104: 345–378
10. Hemalatha MBBS, Bhaskaram P, Qadri SSYH, Kumar PA (1993) Assessment of mild zinc deficiency in children. Nutr Res 13: 115–122
11. Kasarskis E, Schuna A (1980) Serum alkaline phosphatase after treatment of zinc deficiency in humans. Am J Clin Nutr 33: 2609–2612
12. Kirchgessner M, Roth H-P, Weigand E (1976) Biochemical changes in zinc deficiency. In: Trace Elements in Human Health and Disease. Prasad AS, ed. Academic Press, New York 189–225
13. Kirchgessner M, Paulicks BR, Roth H-P (1990) Zink-Funktion, Bedarf, Versorgung und Diagnose. In: Spurenelemente und Ernährung. Wolfram G, Kirchgessner M, Hrsg. Wissenschaftliche Verlagsgesellschaft, Stuttgart 101–121
14. Kirchgessner M (1993) Homeostasis and homeorrhesis in trace element metabolism. In: Trace Elements in Man and Animals – TEMA 8. Anke M, Meissner D, Mills CF, Hrsg. Verlag Media Touristik, Gerstorf 4–21
15. Kruse-Jarres JD (1994) Möglichkeiten und Grenzen der Spurenelementbestimmung in biologischem Material. In: Defizite und Überschüsse an Mengen- und Spurenelementen in der Ernährung. Fresenius W, Brätter P, Liesen H, Dörner K, Hrsg. Harald Schubert Verlag, Leipzig 1–15
16. McMahon RJ, Cousins RJ (1998) Mammalian zinc transporters. J Nutr 128: 667–670
17. Milne DB, Ralston NVC, Wallwork JC (1985) Zinc content of blood cellular components and lymph node and spleen lymphocytes in severely zinc deficient rats. J Nutr 115: 1073–1080
18. Milne DB, Ralston NVC, Wallwork JC (1985) Zinc content of blood: methods for cell separation and analysis evaluated. Clin Chem 31: 65–69
19. Milne DB, Canfield WK, Gallagher SK, Hunt JR, Klevay LM (1987) Ethanol metabolism in postmenopausal women fed a diet marginal in zinc. Am J Clin Nutr 46: 688–693
20. Momcilovic B, Belonje B, Giraux A, Shah BG (1975) Total femur zinc as parameter of choice for a zinc bioassay in rats. Nutr Rep Internat 12: 197–204
21. Naber THJ, Van Den Hamer CJA, Van Den Broek, WJM, Van Tongeren JHM (1992) Zinc uptake by blood cells of rats in zinc deficiency and inflammation. Biol Trace Elem Res 35: 137–152
22. Naber THJ, Heymer F, Van Den Hamer CJA, Van Den Broek WJM, Jansen JBMJ (1994) The invitro uptake of zinc by blood cells in rats with long-term inflammatory stress. Clin Nutr 13: 247–255
23. Pai LH, Prasad AS (1988) Cellular zinc in patients with diabetes mellitus. Nutr Res 8: 889–897
24. Peretz A, Neve J, Jeghers O, Leclercq N, Praet J-P, Vertongen F, Famaey J-P (1991) Interest of zinc determination in leucocyte fractions for the assessment of marginal zinc status. Clin Chim Acta 203: 35–46
25. Prasad AS (1985) Laboratory diagnosing of zinc deficiency. J Am Coll Nutr 4: 591–598
26. Prasad AS, Meftah S, Abdallah J, Kaplan J, Brewer GJ, Bach JF, Dardenne M (1988) Serum thymulin in human zinc deficiency. J Clin Invest 82: 1202–1210
27. Rabbani PI, Prasad AS, Tsai R, Harland BF, Spivey Fox MR (1987) Dietary model for production of experimental zinc deficiency in man. Am J Clin Nutr. 45: 1514–1525

28. Röhrig B, Anke M, Drobner C, Jaritz M, Holzinger S (1998) Zinc intake of German adults with mixed and vegetarian diets. Trace Elements and Electrolytes 15: 81–86

29. Roth H-P, Kirchgessner M (1974) De- und Repletionsstudien an Zink in Knochen und Leber wachsender Ratten. Arch Tierernährg 24: 283–298

30. Roth H-P, Kirchgessner M (1974) Aktivitätsveränderungen verschiedener Dehydrogenasen und der alkalischen Phosphatase im Serum bei Zink-Depletion und -Repletion. Z Tierphysiol Tierernährg u Futtermittelkde 32: 289–296

31. Roth H-P, Kirchgessner M (1979) ^{65}Zn-in vitro Aufnahme der Erythrozyten zur Diagnose von Zn-Mangel. Z Tierphysiol Tierernährg u Futtermittelkde 42: 95–101

32. Roth H-P, Kirchgessner M (1979) Experimentelle Untersuchungen zur Diagnose von marginalem Zinkmangel. Res Exp Med 174: 283–300

33. Roth H-P, Kirchgessner M (1980) Zn-Bindungskapazität des Serums. Ein Parameter zur Diagnose von marginalem Zn-Mangel. Res Exp Med 177: 213–219

34. Roth H-P, Kirchgessner M (1980) Zinkmangel-Diagnose mittels der alkalischen Phosphatase-aktivität im Serum vor und nach einer Zn-Injektion. Zbl Vet Med A 27: 290–297

35. Roth H-P, Kirchgessner M (1994) Influence of zinc deficiency on the osmotic fragility of erythrocyte membranes of force-fed rats. Trace Elements and Electrolytes 11: 46–50

36. Roth H-P, Kirchgessner M (1994) Influence of alimentary zinc deficiency on the concentration of growth hormone (GH), insulin-like growth factor I (IGF-I) and insulin in the serum of force-fed rats. Horm metab Res 26: 404–408

37. Roth H-P, Kirchgessner M (1996) Einfluß von alimentärem Zn-Mangel auf die Konzentration von Wachstumshormon (GH), insulinähnlichem Wachstumsfaktor-1 (IGF-1) und Insulin im Serum von Ratten in Abhängigkeit von der Futteraufnahme. J Anim Physiol a Anim Nutr 76: 180–190

38. Roth H-P, Kirchgessner M (1997) Konzentrationsverlauf an Wachstumshormon, IGF-1, Insulin und C-Peptid in Serum, Hypophyse und Leber von Zn-Mangelratten. J Anim Physiol a Anim Nutr 77: 91–101

39. Ruz M, Cavan KR, Bettger WJ, Thompson LU, Berry M, Gibson RS (1991) Development of a dietary model for the study of marginal zinc deficiency in humans. Evaluation of some biochemical and functional indices of zinc status. Am J Clin Nutr 53: 1–9

40. Ruz M, Cavan KR, Bettger WJ, Gibson RS (1992) Erythrocytes, erythrocyte membranes, neutrophils and platelets as biopsy materials for the assessment of zinc status in humans. Br J Nutr 68: 515–527

41. Smith JC Jr, Babuska L, Ferretti R (1982) Zinc concentration and in vivo uptake of ^{65}zinc in platelets of zinc deficient and control rats. Fed Proc 41: 2991

42. Sullivan VK, Burnett FR, Cousins RJ (1998) Metallothionein expression is increased in monocytes and erythrocytes of young men during zinc supplementation. J Nutr 128: 707–713

43. Taylor CM, Bacon JR, Aggett PJ, Bremner I (1991) Homeostatic regulation of zinc absorption and endogenous losses in zinc-deprived men. Am J Clin Nutr 53: 755–763

44. Thomas EA, Bailey LB, Kauwell GA, Lee D-Y, Cousins RJ (1992) Erythrocyte metallothionein response to dietary zinc in humans. J Nutr 122: 2408–2414

45. Thompson PH (1991) Assessment of zinc status. Proc Nutr Soc 50: 19–28

46. Van Wouwe JP, Veldhuizen M, De Goeij JJM, Van den Hamer CJA (1991) Laboratory assessment of early dietary subclinical zinc deficiency: a model study on weaning rats. Pediatr Res 29: 391–395

47. Weigand E, Kirchgessner M (1980) Total true efficiency of zinc utilization determination and homeostatic dependence upon the zinc supply status in young rats. J Nutr 110: 469–480

Authors' address:

PD Dr. Hans-Peter Roth and Prof. Dr. Dr. h.c. mult. Manfred Kirchgessner
Institut für Ernährungsphysiologie der Technischen Universität München
D-85350 Freising-Weihenstephan, Germany

Dietary supplements and oral feeding in malnutrition*

E. Eisenbart, P. Oster, M. Schuler, G. Schlierf

Geriatrics Centre, Bethanien Hospital, Heidelberg, Germany

Summary

Malnutrition in the elderly should if possible be corrected by the oral route. It represents a particular challenge to relatives, caregivers, and physicians. Because of the individual deficits in each patient, a personal treatment plan has to be devised. Specific measures include optimization of food supply, energy-rich and energy-enriched meals, and liquid nutritional supplements. More general measures include optimization of care during meals and creation of an inviting environment for meal-taking. Success is determined largely by the intensiveness of individual care.

Introduction

Though well documented, the negative effects of malnutrition on general condition, morbidity, and mortality in the elderly receive scant attention in clinical practice. The prognostic importance of various nutritional parameters for health has been demonstrated in a number of studies (3, 5, 20, 26). Malnourished patients have markedly higher morbidity and mortality than adequately nourished patients. Also, increasing evidence has emerged in the last few years that even mild nutritional deficits can have a negative influence on vital functions such as immunity and mental capacity (4).

It is therefore important that malnutrition be avoided and nutritional status improved both in the healthy aging population and in geriatric patients. Firstly, possible causes need to be considered (e.g. physiological causes, effects of diseases and medications, physical, mental, and psychological impairments, socioeconomic factors). There can be no universally valid approach to the treatment of such a highly heterogeneous population as the elderly. Nutritional therapy can be given orally, enterally, or parenterally. Provided the gastrointestinal tract is functional, the oral route is to be preferred. A variety of methods of nutritional therapy are available for use in hospitals, in old peoples and nursing homes, and at home.

* This contribution was translated from German to English by David Playfair, 30 Cheverton Road, London N19 3AY, Great Britain, Email: DavidPlayfair@compuserve.com

Table 1. Measures for oral nutritional therapy

Specific:
- Optimization of food supply (balanced, appropriate, preferred foods that take account of special requirements)
- Energy-rich and energy-enriched foods
- Industrially manufactured dietary supplements

General:
- Optimization of care during meals and of the environment of meal-taking

Specific measures for oral nutritional therapy include consumption of balanced and adequate meals, provision of preferred foods, consumption of food of high nutritional and caloric value, caloric enrichment of standard food, attention to special requirements in terms of the type and consistency of food, and use of liquid nutritional supplements. More general measures relate to the environment of meal-taking and include individual care during meals, provision of special aids, and creation of a suitable and pleasant atmosphere for eating (23) (Table 1).

Though liquid nutritional supplements are reasonably easy to give in the hospital setting, provision of individual nutritional care makes great demands on nurses and kitchen staff, in particular. A number of studies in which the available measures have been combined in various ways have shown that in some cases intervention can bring about substantial improvement in general health and nutritional status.

Optimization of food supply and individual care

Consumption of an adequate and nutritious diet depends upon the availability of a suitable range of foods. This applies both to autonomous elderly people living at home, residents of old peoples and nursing homes, and hospitalized geriatric patients. A balance has to be struck between optimal nutrient composition of the diet and long-established individual habits. This is best achieved by provision of a broad and variable range of foods. Particularly in geriatric patients, but also in basically healthy elderly people, individual requirements are very important in this respect.

People with chewing or swallowing difficulties must be provided with an adequate diet of suitable consistency. They should switch to puréed food only when

Table 2. Aids to eating autonomy for people with functional impairments that affect eating

- Feeding cup with spout
- Cutlery with extra-thick handles
- Fork with one sharpened edge for cutting
- Bent spoon
- Plate with non-slip base
- Cutting board with nails for holding (e.g. bread)

conventional nutritious foods can no longer be adapted to their ability to chew (remove bread crust, peel fruit, use soft foods, etc.). When preparing pured food it is important not just to ensure adequate caloric content, but also to minimize loss of nutrients. To this end, mechanical blending is to be preferred to prolonged cooking (23).

Elderly people who as a result of physical impairments are no longer autonomous in terms of eating should be provided with special aids to help them regain a large measure of autonomy in this respect (Table 2). Consumption of drinks or (thick) liquids such as soup and yoghurt can be considerably facilitated by the use of feeding cups with spouts. Similarly, use of cutlery with extra-thick handles, forks with a sharpened edge for cutting, and bent spoons can help people with only one functional hand to remain autonomous in terms of eating, as can plates with a non-slip base and cutting boards fitted with nails for holding a slice of bread in place (23).

The influence of mental impairments on food consumption is determined by the nature and extent of the impairment. Like patients with physical impairments, these patients require individualized care. It is important to ensure that meals are taken regularly, special preferences are taken into account, and use is made of appropriate aids.

Individual care is especially important in patients with eating apraxia, e.g. as a result of a stroke. These patients must be given help with meals, if possible as part of their occupational therapy.

In addition to the points mentioned above, the social aspects of eating are of particular importance to elderly people.

A study conducted at the Bethanien Hospital in Heidelberg (10) investigated the effects of three weeks of individual nutritional care by a dietitian on the food intake and nutritional state of undernourished female geriatric patients. Within the limits of the type of food prescribed in the individual case and the range of foods available at the hospital, the 20 patients in the intervention group were allowed to eat whatever they wished and were provided with additional high-energy foods in accordance with their likes and dislikes. They were given intensive care at meals in the form of help with cutting and eating, motivation, and company. The control group received standard dietary care. Success was assessed via energy intake and a number of nutrition-dependent blood parameters. The intervention group showed a mean increase in energy intake of 120 kcal (502 kJ) per day. Although there were no statistically significant changes in body weight or nutrition-dependent blood parameters during the three-week period of the study, a tendency to an increase in weight was seen. The control group showed a further loss of weight during the study, the median weight of the patients at the end of the study being 500 g less than that of the patients in the intervention group. Although the results achieved in this relatively short period were not statistically significant, they do suggest that more intensive attention and support at mealtimes can lead to an improvement in food intake and thus in the long term to an improvement in nutritional condition. This impression has been confirmed in other studies on dependent elderly nursing home patients given assistance with meals. The nutrient intake of such patients was found to be markedly higher than that of apparently independent patients (9, 18). The fact that dietary behaviour is also influenced by physical environment was confirmed by Elmstahl et al. (8) in a study on 16 residents of a geriatric long-term-care home. Over a period of 16 weeks the dining room was fitted out in 1940s style and the food provided in a way that allowed the patients to serve themselves. In this altered environment energy and protein intake rose by about 25 %. During the period of the study the patients' mean daily energy intake showed a significant rise of 340 kcal (1.4 MJ) from its baseline level of 1379 kcal (5.8 MJ). A number of nutrition-dependent blood parameters (folate, creatinine, retinol) also rose significantly during the study.

Energy-rich and energy-enriched food

To date few studies have been conducted on the use of energy-rich and energy-enriched food in undernourished elderly people. Here too, however, there is much potential for improving nutrition. Winograd & Brown (28) succeeded in reawakening appetite and interest in food in undernourished patients with a poor appetite by providing a greater range of the patients' favourite sweets. They then increased the range of standard foods, which thereupon came to be increasingly accepted by the patients. In this way they achieved marked improvements in the patients' clinical course, general condition, and weight development (increases of up to 9 kg in two months) and in a number of nutrition-dependent blood parameters (e.g. albumin level rose by up to 50 %). In another study (21), standard foods were enriched with taste-neutral supplements. This considerably increased the nutritional value and caloric density of drinks and meals. Mean daily energy intake was increased by 1200 kcal (5 MJ), serum albumin and transferrin levels rose, and most patients showed a positive nitrogen balance after the intervention.

Liquid nutritional supplements

In addition to nutritional therapy in the form of standard foods and dishes, the food industry offers a variety of nutritional supplements aimed at optimizing daily energy and nutrient intake. These supplements are supplied by various manufacturers in various types of pack in the form of instantly soluble powder or as liquid or creamy ready-to-consume products. Ready-to-drink liquid nutritional supplements are supplied in bottles, Tetrapacks, or cartons of 175 to 250 ml. A variety of sweet and savoury tastes and both milk- and juice-based sweet products are available. These various liquid nutritional supplements contain defined amounts of nutrients in the form of high molecular weight complex carbohydrates, proteins, and fats. The standard forms have an energy content of 1 kcal (4.2 kJ) per ml and consist of 14–20 % protein, 25–35 % fat, and 50–60 % carbohydrates. The vitamin and mineral content is generally such that 2000 ml of liquid supplies the daily requirements of all nutrients. Also available are a number of high-caloric variants containing up to 1.6 kcal/ml and protein-rich variants in which up to 35 % of the energy content is supplied by protein.

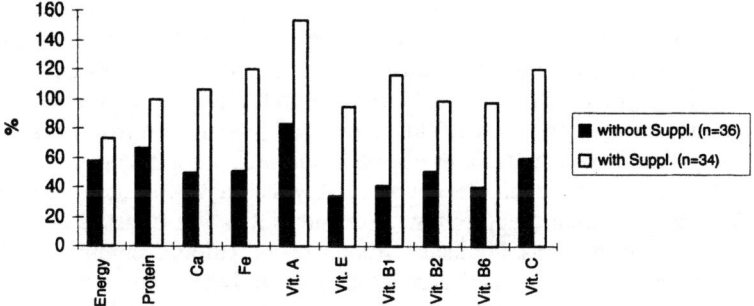

Fig. 1. Mean daily nutrient uptake of hospitalized undernourished female geriatric patients without (n = 36) and with (n = 34) nutritional supplementation: percentage satisfaction of DGE* 1991 recommended daily allowances (7) (Hübsch et al. 1994). *Deutsche Gesellschaft für Ernährung (German Nutrition Association).

Liquid nutritional supplements represent an important option for oral nutritional therapy in undernourished patients. A large number of studies have shown that consumption of energy- and nutrient-rich liquid food can improve nutrient intake (1, 6, 8, 15, 12, 13, 19, 22, 25) and nutritional condition as assessed by anthropometric and biochemical parameters (1, 6, 8, 12, 14, 15, 17, 21), reduce mortality (14), and shorten hospitalization times (2, 6).

Thus, in a pilot study conducted at the Bethanien Hospital in Heidelberg (13) it was shown that energy and nutrient intake can be increased by oral supplementation without reduction in food intake via standard hospital food. In a subsequent randomized controlled study (12), use of a mean dose of 193 ml (232 kcal/970 kJ) of liquid supplement led to increases in energy and nutrient intake as compared with a control group (n = 36) not given the supplement. Thanks to the high nutrient density of the supplement, the recommended dietary allowances (7) for healthy elderly people were achieved in the case of nearly all nutrients in the group given the supplement (n = 34) (Fig. 1). This group also showed positive effects in terms of bodily composition, vitamin status (blood levels), and need for nursing care. During the period of hospitalization the patients' ADL score (16) rose by a mean of 20 points in the subgroup with good acceptance of the supplement (SG+), remained the same in the subgroup with poor acceptance of the supplement (SG-), and rose by a mean of 5 points in the control group. Patients who continued to receive the supplement for six months after discharge from hospital showed a further improvement in degree of autonomy, the ADL score rising by a further 5 points in the SG+ subgroup, rising by 2.5 points in the control subgroup, and falling by 10 points in the SG- subgroup (25).

In a Swiss study on geriatric patients with a fractured neck of the femur (6), use of liquid nutritional supplements reduced the complication rate, rehabilitation time, and mortality rate as compared with a control group not given the supplements (n = 32). During their period of hospitalization (mean 32 days) the patients in the group given the supplement (n = 27) received 250 ml (254 kcal/1067 kJ) of supplement per day. In another study (14), oral nutritional supplementation of geriatric patients in long-term care led to maintenance or improvement in nutritional status and to a reduction in mortality. The supplemented group (n = 197) received 400 ml (400 kcal/1680 kJ) of liquid nutritional supplement per day in addition to the standard hospital food. The nutritional status of the supplemented and the control group (n = 238) was assessed at the start of the study and after 26 weeks.

One problem that commonly arises with the use of liquid nutritional supplements is that of acceptance. The mere act of placing a nutritional supplement on the patient's bedside table or elsewhere in his/her room is generally not in itself sufficient to ensure that the supplement will actually be taken on a regular basis. With many patients, appropriate care and motivation is just as important here as with standard meals. Published studies on nutritional supplementation contain discrepant data on levels of acceptance. In a study by Delmi et al. (6), the 250 ml of liquid nutritional supplement that was provided was well tolerated and reportedly consumed in its entirety. Other studies (11, 27) have reported poor or very poor acceptance of supplements by quite a high proportion of study participants. Williams et al. (27) took this factor into account by separately investigating not just a control group (n = 19) and a supplemented group (n = 19), but also a non-compliance group (n = 11). Average daily consumption of supplement was 1.6 packets (400 kcal/1680 kJ) in the group as a whole but only 20–100 ml in the patients with poor acceptance. As expected, only the group with good acceptance benefited from the supplement. In a study by Hübsch (11), 400 ml of liquid nutritional supplement was provided per day. Of the total of 35 patients investigated, nine were found to have poor compliance (consumption < 133 ml/day), 21 to have fair compliance (consumption 133–266 ml/day), and five to have good compliance (consumption > 266 ml/day). Average consumption of supplement in the group as a whole was 200 ml/day. In this study also, the success of nutritional supplementation increased with increasing consumption. Therefore, when liquid nutritional supplements are used for oral nutritional therapy, every effort should be made to ensure regular and high consumption.

In order to improve the acceptance of liquid nutritional supplements in the elderly, a variety of tastes should be provided via the use of different products (24). One such possibility is to combine sweet and savoury variants. Volkert et al. (25) offered their patients a savoury soup in the morning and a milk-based sweet drink in the afternoon.

For some time now not only milk-based, but also juice-based, sweet drinks have been available. These contain no milk protein and are therefore also suitable for patients with milk protein intolerance. Especially when cool, they are also more refreshing than milk-based drinks. In an as-yet unpublished study by the present authors, geriatric patients given the choice of a juice-based or a milk-based variant chose the former more often (34 vs. 25). Nevertheless, the amount consumed and the resulting energy intake were somewhat less with fruit juice than with milk-based drinks (mean 159 ml/197 kcal and 220 ml/232 kcal, respectively). This may have been partly due to the fact that the juice-based drinks were often diluted with water. As some patients consumed both types of supplement, the mean energy intake of the whole group attributable to the liquid nutritional supplements was 250 kcal/day, a level slightly higher than that found in the studies by Jakobeit (13) and Hübsch et al. (12) referred to above. In any case, fruit-based drinks represent a useful addition to the available range of liquid nutritional supplements.

References

1. Banerjee AK, Brocklehurst JC, Wainwright H, Swindell R (1978) Nutritional status of long-stay geriatric in-patients: effects of a food supplement (Complan). Age and Aging 7: 237–243
2. Bastow MD, Rawlings J, Allison SP (1983) Benefits of supplementary tube feeding after fractured neck of femur: A randomised controlled trial. Br Med J 287: 1589–1592
3. Bienia R, Ratcliff S, Barbour GL, Kummer M (1982) Malnutrition in the hospitalized geriatric patient. J Am Geriatr Soc 30: 433–436
4. Buzina R, Bates CJ, van der Beek J et al. (1989) Workshop on functional significance of mild-to-moderate malnutrition. Am J Clin Nutr 50: 172–176
5. Constans T, Bacq Y, Bréchot JF, Guilmot JL, Choutet P, Lamisse F (1992) Protein-energy malnutrition in elderly medical patients. J Am Geriatr Soc 40: 263–268
6. Delmi M, Rapin CH, Benoga JM, Delmas PD, Vasey H (1990) Dietary supplementation in elderly patients with fractured neck of femur. Lancet 335: 1013–1016
7. Deutsche Gesellschaft für Ernährung (1991) Empfehlungen für die Nährstoffzufuhr. 5. Überarbeitung. Umschau Verlag, Frankfurt
8. Elmstahl S, Steen B (1987) Hospital nutrition in geriatric long-term care medicine: II. Effects of dietary supplements. Age and Aging 16: 73–80
9. Evans E, Stock AL (1971) Dietary intake of geriatric patients in hospital. Nutr Metab 13: 21–35
10. Göhner M (1995) Verbesserung der Ernährungssituation geriatrischer Patientinnen mit Risikofaktoren für Unterernährung. Diplomarbeit, University of Hohenheim
11. Hübsch S (1995) Auswirkungen der Ernährungstherapie mit flüssiger Zusatznahrung auf Nahrungsaufnahme, Ernährungsstatus und klinischen Verlauf bei mangelernährten geriatrischen Patienten. Dissertation, University of Hohenheim
12. Hübsch S, Volkert D, Oster P, Schlierf G (1994) Möglichkeiten und Grenzen der Anwendung flüssiger Nährstoffkonzentrate in der Therapie der Mangelernährung geriatrischer Patienten. Akt Ernähr Med 19: 109–114
13. Jakobeit G (1991) Einfluß oraler Nahrungssupplementation auf die Nährstoffzufuhr unterernährter geriatrischer Patientinnen. Inaugural Dissertation, University of Heidelberg
14. Larsson J, Unosson M, Ek AC, Nilsson L, Thorslund S, Bjurulf P (1990) Effect of dietary supplement on nutritional status and clinical outcome in 501 geriatric patients – a randomised study. Clin Nutr 9: 179–184
15. Lipschitz DA, Mitchell CO, Steele RW, Milton KY (1985) Nutritional evaluation and supplementation of elderly subjects participating in a ìmeals on wheelsî program. J Paret Ent Nutr 9: 343–347
16. Mahoney F, Barthel D (1965) Functional evaluation: The Barthel Index. Md State Med J 14: 61–65
17. McEvoy AW, James OFW (1982) The effect of a dietary supplement (Build-up) on nutritional status in hospitalized elderly patients. Hum Nutr Appl Nutr 36A: 374–376
18. Nguyen NH, Flint DM, Prinsley DM, Wahlqvist ML (1985) Nutrient intakes of dependent and apparently independent nursing home patients. Hum Nutr Appl Nutr 39A: 333–338
19. Ovesen L (1992) The effect of a supplement which is nutrient dense compared to standard concentration on the total nutritional intake of anorectic patients. Clin Nutr 11: 154–157
20. Sullivan DH, Walls TC, Lipschitz DA (1991) Protein-energy undernutrition and the risk of mortality within 1 y of hospital discharge in a select population of geriatric rehabilitation patients. Am J Clin Nutr 53: 599–605
21. Tomaiolo PP, Enman S, Kraus V (1981) Preventing and treating malnutrition in the elderly. J Parent Ent Nutr 5: 46–48
22. Unosson M, Larsson K, Ek AC, Bjurulf P (1992) Effects of dietary supplement on functional condition and clinical outcome measured with a modified Norton scale. Clin Nutr 11: 134–139
23. Volkert D (1997) Ernährung im Alter. UTB für Wissenschaft, Quelle & Meyer Wiesbaden, 247–257

24. Volkert D (1997) Wann sind Nahrungssupplemente sinnvoll? Home Care 5 (1): 6–8
25. Volkert D, Hübsch S, Oster P, Schlierf G (1996) Nutritional support and functional status in undernourished geriatric patients during hospitalization and 6 months follow-up. Aging Clin Exp Res 8: 386–395
26. Volkert D, Kruse W, Oster P, Schlierf G (1992) Malnutrition in geriatric patients: diagnostic and prognostic significance of nutritional parameters. Ann Nutr Metab 36: 97–112
27. Williams CM, Driver LT, Older J, Dickerson JWT (1989) A controlled trial of sip-feed supplements in elderly orthopaedic patients. Eur J Clin Nutr 43: 267–274
28. Winograd CH, Brown EM (1990) Aggressive oral refeeding in hospitalized patients. Am J Clin Nutr 52: 967–968

Author's address:

Dipl. oec. troph. Eva Eisenbart
Prof. Dr. med. Peter Oster
Dr. med. Matthias Schuler
Prof. Dr. med. Günter Schlierf
Bethanien-Krankenhaus, Geriatrisches Zentrum
Rohrbacher Str. 149
D-69126 Heidelberg, Germany

Tube feeding in malnutrition*

A. Jordan, W. F. Caspary, J. Stein

Zentrum der Inneren Medizin, Klinikum der Johann Wolfgang Goethe-Universität Frankfurt, Frankfurt, Germany

Summary

Malnutrition is very common in geriatric patients, with a cited prevalence of 30 to 60 %. Therefore, nutritional support via nasogastric or percutaneous tubes is frequently indicated. As percutaneous endoscopic gastrostomy (PEG) has several advantages over nasogastric tube feeding including reduced risk of tube dislodgement and blockage and higher patient acceptance, it has become the method of choice for enteral tube feeding. Complication rates are low provided that guidelines for enteral tube feeding are observed. Early home enteral nutrition enhances patients' quality of life.

Introduction

Malnutrition is a very common problem in geriatric patients, with a cited prevalence of 30 to 60 % (1, 20). Poor nutritional status has a negative impact on the patient's morbidity, mortality, and quality of life. Manifest malnutrition calls for intensive nutritional support. In the interests of their mental and social well-being, geriatric patients should of course be encouraged to consume food via the natural route for as long as possible; however, once nutritional requirements can no longer be met by oral food intake, either supportive or exclusively "artificial" nutritional therapy is required.

Indications

The objective of enteral nutrition is to treat or prevent malnutrition in patients with inadequate oral food intake. Therefore there is a broad range of indications for initiation of tube feeding in geriatric patients:

---

* This contribution was translated from German to English by David Playfair, 30 Cheverton Road, London N19 3AY, Great Britain, Email: DavidPlayfair@compuserve.com

▶ Oncological diseases (cancerous cachexia, stenosing ENT tumours, tumours of the upper gastrointestinal tract)
▶ Neurological diseases (cerebrovascular accident, persistent vegetative state, brain tumours, Parkinson's disease)
▶ Neuropsychiatric diseases (senile dementia, depression, neurosis, psychosis)

The decision to initiate intensive nutritional therapy calls for a precise evaluation of the advantages and disadvantages of tube feeding to the patient concerned. The value of enteral nutrition in terms of the nutritional condition of malnourished patients is beyond question; however it must not be forgotten that tube feeding constitutes a considerable intrusion into the patients life and illness. Therefore, in addition to the medical indication for tube feeding, ethical considerations such as the patient's autonomy and quality of life and the wishes of the patient and his/her family and caregivers should be included into the decision-making process (23).

Techniques

Enteral nutrition can be achieved via a number of different methods whose appropriateness in the individual patient depends upon the indication, the predicted duration of the need for enteral feeding, and organ-specific considerations.

Transnasal tubes

The simplest method of gaining access to the gastrointestinal tract is via transnasal tube systems. A tube is passed through the nose and advanced into the stomach, duodenum, or jejunum. Correct placement must be verified by means of a radiograph. Placement in the distal duodenum or in the jejunum is via radiological or endoscopic techniques.

Nasal tubes are of only limited usefulness for long-term feeding, as they induce a foreign-body sensation in the pharynx, can cause reflux oesophagitis and pressure ulcers, and have a tendency to dislodge (13). They can also be a psychological burden to the patient, as the visible presence of the tube advertises the fact that the patient is ill. This can be disadvantageous especially in ambulant patients and in social settings. Enteral feeding via transnasal tubes is often poorly tolerated by geriatric patients with acute confusional states. The need for repeated insertion of tubes following forcible removal by the patient is very demanding on nursing staff. Moreover, long-term restraint of the patient is often required (5). Nasal tubes are unsuitable for patients with potentially reversible dysphagia – in most cases due to a cerebrovascular accident – who are to undergo orofacial therapy for their dysphagia. The presence of a nasal tube interferes to a large extent with swallowing training (18). For all these reasons nasal tubes are generally used only for short-term enteral feeding and in situations in which other methods of enteral feeding are contraindicated.

Where feeding via a transnasal tube is indicated, narrow-lumen (Charrier 8), tissue-friendly polyurethane or silicone rubber tubes with suitable bandaging sets should be used in order to prevent dislodgement and slippage.

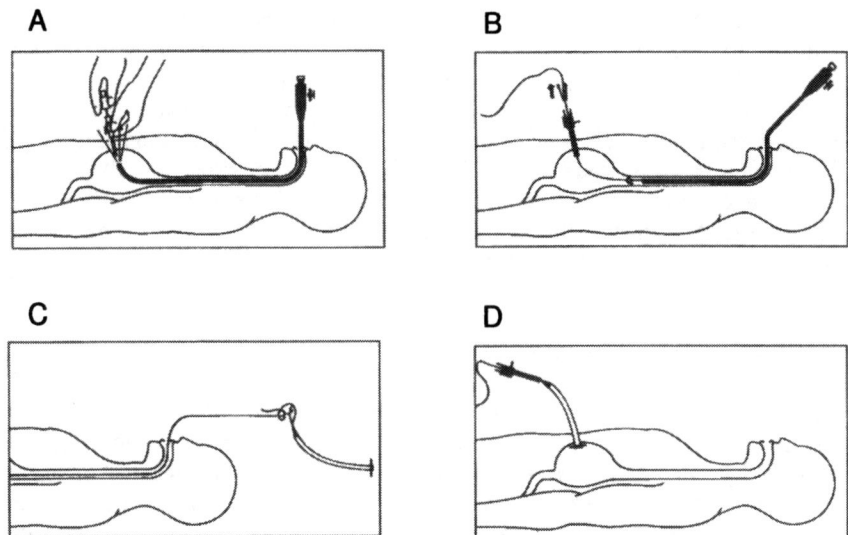

Fig. 1. Placement of a percutaneous endoscopic gastrostomy (PEG) using the thread pull-through method.
A. The gastroscope is introduced into the stomach and an adequate amount of air is insufflated. After administration of local anaesthetic to all layers of the stomach wall, a puncture needle through which a guide thread has been passed is advanced from the exterior in the region of the diaphanoscopy. **B.** With the aid of forceps, the guide thread is withdrawn from the stomach together with the gastroscope. **C.** The proximal end of the thread is attached to the catheter. **D.** The tube is pulled through the stomach wall to the exterior by gentle traction on the distal end of the thread until the retaining disc abuts against the inside of the stomach wall.

Percutaneous endoscopic gastrostomy (PEG)

One technique that circumvents the upper aerodigestive tract is percutaneous endoscopic gastrostomy (PEG). Placement is performed via a brief endoscopic procedure under local anaesthesia (14) (Fig. 1). The tube is generally placed in the stomach. Suitable double-lumen tubes can be placed in the intestine. PEG has proved to be safe, relatively complication-free, practicable, and well tolerated by patients (16, 19). The mortality related to the technique is 0.5 %. Serious complications such as peristomal leakage with peritonitis, necrotizing fasciitis of the anterior abdominal wall, and gastric bleeding are rare (< 1 %). The most frequent complication of PEG is peristomal wound infection; the frequency of which is cited in the literature at between 3 and 30 % (6, 11, 16). Regular skin and stomal care is required if local infection is to be prevented. Also important is bandaging technique. In a comparative study, Chung (1990) showed that excessive traction on the gastrostomy tube significantly increases the rate of local infection (2). Antibiotic prophylaxis is recommended for patients with impaired immune function; however the need for routine antibiotic prophylaxis prior to PEG placement is disputed (7, 8). In one study, administration of 1 g of a cephalosporin 30 min before PEG placement reduced the incidence of peristomal wound infection from 29 % to 7 % (7).

PEG has proved to be the method of choice for longer-term enteral nutritional support provided that the contraindications to its use are observed. As stated above, it has a series of advantages over transnasal feeding tubes.

Percutaneous gastric feeding can be achieved using replaceable "buttons" that are inserted in an established gastrostomy. These have the advantage that they can be inserted and removed without the need for further gastroscopy. They also have a very flat external retaining disc and are attached to the feeding system via a safety connector. They thus allow the patient great freedom of movement and scarcely interfere with any kind of activity.

Fine-needle-catheter jejunostomy (FCJ)

Another method of enteral feeding is fine-needle-catheter jejunostomy (FCJ). FCJs are generally inserted only in association with abdominal surgery. They are technically easy to insert and offer patients the same advantages as PEG in terms of comfort and low complication rates. The complication rate of FCJ insertion is cited in the literature at less than 1 %. The most frequent serious complication is dislodgement of the catheter (11, 22).

Enteral feeding products

Industrially manufactured balanced diets, the composition of which is in accordance with the recommendations of the German Nutrition Association (DGE), are available for enteral feeding. These diets, which can be drunk or administered by tube, can be classified as either high molecular weight, nutrient-defined diets (NDDs) or low molecular weight, chemically-defined diets (CDDs) (Table 1).

Chemically defined diets (CDDs) are used in patients with impaired digestion and absorption. Their principal nutrients are enzymatically predigested to an extent that renders them directly absorbable (4). The protein component consists of protein hydrolysates (oligopeptides). Carbohydrates are present in the form of oligosaccharides, and the fat component contains a high proportion of medium-chain-triglyceride (MCT) fats (12, 17). The fat component of CDDs is somewhat reduced (15–20 %) and the carbohydrate component correspondingly increased (60–70 %) (3).

Standard NDDs generally contain 15–20 % protein, 25–35 % fat, and 45–55 % carbohydrate. Their principal nutrients are high-quality native protein (mostly milk and soya protein), oligo- and polysaccharides (maltodextrin), and plant oils in the form of triglycerides with long-chain fatty acids (sunflower, soya, and safflower oils). The use of NDDs thus presupposes essentially intact digestive and absorptive function (4). Special diets are available for use in patients with diabetes mellitus or impaired liver or renal function.

Table 1. Types of formula diet for enteral nutrition

Nutrient-defined diets (NDDs)	
High molecular weight substrates	
1. Standard diet:	Intact protein, poly- & oligosaccharides, long-chain triglycerides
	1 kcal/ml
	Roughage-free
2. Modified NDD:	Roughage-containing
	Energy density > 1.5 kcal/ml
	Protein content > 20 % of total energy
	Medium-chain triglycerides
	Increased content of branched-chain amino acids
	High fat content (> 45 % of total energy)
	Fatty acid-modified (omega-3 fatty acids)
	Glutamine-containing
Chemically defined diets (CDDs)	
Low molecular weight substrates	
1. Oligopeptide diet:	Oligopeptides, oligo- & monosaccharides, medium-chain triglycerides
	1 kcal/ml
	Roughage-free
2. Modified CDD:	Disease-adapted by modification of carbohydrate, fat, or protein component

Forms of administration

The form of administration to be used depends upon the location of the end of the tube, the disease from which the patient suffers, and the type of diet to be given. Where gastric function is unimpaired, the food can be given via a gastric tube. This has the advantage that the reservoir function of the stomach is retained and the contents of the stomach pass to the small intestine in portions, permitting intermittent administration of the food with the aid of gravity. This is the more physiological form of tube feeding. Intermittent feeding can have side effects such as regurgitation, aspiration, and dumping symptoms, especially if the food is given too rapidly and is too cold when given.

Placement of the feeding tube in the upper small intestine is indicated in patients with stenotic processes of the pyloric region or intestine, unconscious patients and patients with impaired consciousness (because of the risk of aspiration), and patients with disturbances of gastric emptying such as diabetic gastroparesis. Placement of the tube in the intestine necessitates continuous pump-assisted administration of the food (17).

Tube-feeding must be established gradually and adapted in accordance with the individual tolerance of the patient. The adaptation phase is shorter with gastric than with intestinal administration. The rate of administration should be increased only after a 24-hour period of administration without complications. When an increase in administration rate leads to the appearance of symptoms, the rate should be reduced (9).

Complications of enteral feeding

The frequency of complications of enteral feeding varies considerably in accordance with the method and site of administration, the composition of the formula diet used, and the severity of the underlying disease. Also important is the experience of the clinician. The complication rate can be reduced by careful observance of guidelines on tube feeding including those relating to food composition, administration rate, portion size, food temperature, and supervision of the patient. The most common complications of enteral feeding are gastrointestinal in origin, e.g. diarrhoea, nausea and/or vomiting, constipation, and feelings of fullness (9, 11, 12). If complications occur, the cause must first be identified. It must be remembered that gastrointestinal symptoms can be caused not just by enteral feeding itself, but

Table 2. Gastrointestinal complications of enteral nutrition – causes, prevention, treatment

Complication	Cause	Prevention/treatment
Diarrhoea	Too rapid increase in amount of food per day	Observe adaptation phase
	Too rapid administration of food	Reduce/control administration rate
	Food too cold	Increase to room temperature
	Osmolarity too high (> 300 mosm)	Use isotonic feeding solution, initially dilute hyperosmolar feeding solutions
	Lactose intolerance	Use low-lactose or lactose-free diet
	Fat malabsorption	Use low-fat or MCT-containing diet
	Hypoalbuminaemia	Use chemically defined diet and/or feed parenterally until absorptive capacity of small intestine restored
	Long-term antibiotic therapy	Review medications / give antidiarrhoeals
	Chemotherapy/radiotherapy	Antidiarrhoeals
Nausea/vomiting	Too rapid administration of food	Reduce/control administration rate
	Contamination of food, delivery equipment	Change delivery equipment every 24 hours, handle administration systems hygienically, keep opened bottles of formula no more than 24 hours in refrigerator
Cramps/bloating	Too rapid administration of food	Reduce/control administration rate
	Lactose intolerance	Use low-lactose or lactose-free diet
	Fat malabsorption	Use low-fat or MCT-containing diet
Regurgitation/aspiration	Gastric retention	Reduce administration rate, prefer duodenal tube, incline patient during food administration
Constipation	Inadequate fluid intake	Increase fluid intake, check fluid balance
	Roughage intake too low	Use roughage-containing formula

also by the underlying disease or by therapeutic measures such as antibiotic therapy, chemotherapy, or radiotherapy.

The incidence of diarrhoea in association with enteral feeding is 2–68 %, depending on the definition of diarrhoea used. Formed or doughy stools should not be described as diarrhoea even if they are passed six or seven times a day. Diarrhoea can be due to the composition or the method or rate of administration of the formula diet or to medications or infections. Sorbitol-containing medications can cause diarrhoea, as can antibiotics (by altering the intestinal flora and favouring the growth of Clostridium difficile). Table 2 summarizes the specific complications of enteral feeding and the treatment and prevention of these.

A possible complication in geriatric patients with impaired level of consciousness is aspiration of administered food. Patients who experience feelings of fullness and show a tendency to regurgitation and aspiration should be placed in an inclined position (about 30°) during and after administration of food and should be fed at a slower rate. If symptoms are severe, consideration should be given to moving the tube from a gastric to a duodenal position.

Home enteral nutrition

Until recently, enteral nutrition was restricted to hospitals and nursing homes. Now, however, patients can, after successful inpatient treatment and appropriate training, feed themselves by the enteral route at home. The return to the patient's familiar environment brings with it a significant improvement in quality of life, and this in turn usually has a positive influence on the patients general health.

Success with ambulant enteral feeding depends critically upon careful training of patients and their relatives and caregivers and the existence of an effective ambulant care system (nurse, physician, health insurance fund, pharmacy, formula diet manufacturer). Also important for a smooth transition of patients from the hospital to the domestic environment is the hospital-based nutrition team responsible for training patients and their families and organizing ambulant nutritional therapy (21).

References

1. Adil A, Abbasi MD, Rudman D (1994) Undernutrition in the nursing home: prevalence, consequences, causes and prevention. Nutr Rev 52: 113–120
2. Chung RS, Schertzer M (1990) Pathogenesis of complications of percutaneous endoscopic gastrostomy. A lesson in surgical principles. Am Surg 56: 134–137
3. Hohner E, Prinz A (1993) Aktuelle Aspekte der enteralen Ernährung. Ernährungs-Umschau 40: 4–10
4. Höllwarth I, Schlag P (1990) Leitfaden der enteralen Ernährung. Kohlhammer, Stuttgart, Berlin, Cologne
5. Honneth J, Nehen HG (1990) PEG – effiziente Methode für die enterale Langzeiternährung. Geriatrie Praxis 10: 56–61
6. Hull MA, Rawlings J, Murray FE et al. (1993) Audit of outcome of long-term enteral nutrition by percutaneous endoscopic gastrostomy. Lancet 341: 869–872

7. Jain NK, Larson DE, Schroeder KW et al. (1987) Antibiotic prophylaxis for percutaneous endoscopic gastrostomy. Ann Int Med 107: 824–828

8. Jonas SK, Neimark S, Panwalker AP (1985) Effect of antibiotic prophylaxis in percutaneous endoscopic gastrostomy. Am J Gastroenterol 80: 438–441

9. Jordan, A, Emde A, Markus A, Caspary WF, Stein J (1997) Enterale Ernährung tumorkranker Patienten. Akt Ernähr Med 22: 4–8

10. Jordan A, Stein J (1997) Pathophysiologie der Tumorkachexie. Ernährungs-Umschau 44: 250–254

11. Jordan A, Stein J (1997) Komplikationen bei Tumorpatienten mit enteraler Langzeiternährung. Ernährungs-Umschau 44: 289–293

12. Jordan A, Stein J, Caspary WF (1998) Ambulante parenterale und enterale Ernährung. In: Moderne Infusionstherapie. Künstliche Ernährung (W. Harig, ed.), 8th edn. Zuckschwerdt Verlag (in print)

13. Kemen M, Homann HH, Senkal M, Zumtobel V (1994) Die Bedeutung der postoperativen enteralen Ernährung. Chirurg Gastroenterol 10: 198–201

14. Keymling M (1989) Perkutane endoskopisch kontrollierte Gastrostomie. Z Gastroent 27 (Suppl 2): 65–68

15. Kolb S, Ruppin H, Sailer D, Iro H, Fietkau R, Thiel HJ (1988) Enterale Langzeiternährung über perkutane, endoskopisch kontrolliert plazierte Gastrostomiesonden – Ergebnisse bei 108 vorwiegend ambulant betreuten Patienten. Med Klin 83: 96–99

16. Larson DE, Burton DD, Schroeder KW, DiMagno EP (1987) Percutaneous endoscopic gastrostomy: Indications, success, complications, and mortality in 314 consecutive patients. Gastroenterology 93: 48–52

17. Manegold BC, Mechtersheimer U, Jung M (1987) Applikationsformen zur enteralen Sondenernährung – ein Überblick. Med Welt 38: 17–25

18. Michaelis M (1997) Die PEG in der Geriatrie: Schwere Essprobleme lassen sich lösen. Geriatrie Praxis 7–8: 39–41

19. Moran BJ, Taylor MB, Johnson CD (1990) Percutaneous endoscopic gastrostomy. Br J Surg 77: 858–862

20. Morley JE, Glick Z, Rubenstein IZ (1990) Geriatric nutrition: a comprehensive review. New York, Raven Press

21. Rabast U, Heskamp R, Hinge J (1986) Aufgaben eines Ernährungsteams bei der Sondenernährung. Ernährungs-Umschau 33 (Sonderheft): S472–S477

22. Vestweber KH, Eypasch E, Paul A, Bode C, Troidl H (1989) Feinnadel-Katheter-Jejunostomie. Z Gastroenterol 27 (Suppl 2): 69–72

23. Watts DT, Cassel CK, Hickam DH (1986) Nurses' and physicians' attitudes towards tubefeeding decisions in long-term care. J Am Geriatr Soc 34: 607–611

Author's address:

Prof. Dr. W. F. Caspary
Medizinische Klinik II
Zentrum der Inneren Medizin
Klinikum der Johann Wolfgang Goethe-Universität Frankfurt
Theodor-Stern-Kai 7
60590 Frankfurt, Germany

Zinc: pathophysiologic effects, nutritional deficiency, and effects of supplementation in older people – a review

A. Abbasi, K. Shetty

Department of Medicine, Medical College of Wisconsin, Milwaukee, WI, USA

Summary

Zinc is an essential micronutrient. Several studies have shown that zinc deficiency is common in older people. Zinc has been extensively studied with regard to its role in wound healing, infections, immune system, cardiovascular disease, and several other medical conditions. Several investigators have published intervention studies using zinc supplements in older people with favorable outcomes. This paper will briefly review the pathophysicologic effects of zinc, nutritional deficiency, and effects of zinc supplementation in older people.

Introduction

Several studies have shown wide variation in the nutritional status of older people (1, 19). Nutritional surveys of the community-dwelling older people have shown that the suboptimal essential nutrient status is not uncommon in this age group (60 years and older). The surveys of institutionalized older people have consistently shown a less favorable picture as compared to the community-dwelling, independent older people (1). In the institutionalized older people, intake for both calories and proteins are frequently low. Up to 50 % of the subjects are suboptimal in body weight, midarm muscle circumference, and serum albumin level, indicating wide-spread protein calorie undernutrition.

Due to the declining caloric requirements with age and therefore a reduced food intake, the risk of micronutrient deficiencies increases in older people, unless the nutrient density of the diet is increased. This may explain the common occurance of micronutirent deficiency in older people, especially frail institutionalized older people, as discussed earlier in this paper.

The ingested food needs to be properly digested for liberation and optimum utilization of the minerals and trace elements present in the diet. The hydrolysis of bonds between minerals and macronutrients of the diet require an acidic pH, which liberates the elements and maintains them in soluble form. Some published reports have shown that atrophic gastritis with impaired gastric acid production may be present in up to one third of older people (18). An acid pH is needed to facilitate absorption of cationic elements such as calcium, chromium, copper, iron, manganese, and zinc. The high prevalance of atrophic gastritis in older people, further increases the risk of mineral and trace element deficiency in this population.

Zinc: an essential nutrient

Zinc is an essential micronutrient. Zinc is needed for DNA synthesis, cell division, and protein synthesis. There are approximately 300 zinc containing enzymes known to us today. It is believed that several hundred zinc containing nucleoproteins may be involved in gene expression of various proteins.

Pathophysiologic effects of zinc

Wound healing

Several investigators have demonstrated the beneficial effects of zinc on wound healing (2, 8). It has been found that patients with leg ulcers often have reduced serum zinc levels (9). Several investigators have studied the effect of zinc supplement on the healing of leg ulcers. Hallbrook and Lanner (13) have shown that zinc supplementation was beneficial in patients with leg ulcers who had low serum zinc level. There are, however, some published reports which have shown no benefit from oral zinc supplement in patients with leg ulcers (23).

Several studies using the animal model have shown beneficial effects of topical zinc in leg ulcers (21, 22) . The published reports in human subjects with leg ulcers using topical zinc are less convincing. Agren (2) randomized 37 subjects with leg ulcers to zinc oxide or placebo treatment. At the end of eight weeks, the success rate (using predetermined criteria) was significantly higher ($P < 0.05$) for the zinc vs the placebo group (83 % vs 42 %). In this study, the mean serum zinc levels was significantly lower in patients with leg ulcers, as compared to the age-matched controls. The investigator, however, found no correlation between serum zinc level and wound healing.

Immune system

The immune function declines with advancing age as evident from thymic atrophy, decreased delayed type hypersensitivity responses, and reduced responses to antigenic and mitogenic stimuli. One consistent observation, in most studies, has been a decline in T cell function. Several studies have found anergy, selective decline in CD4 T lymphocytes (helper cells), decreased natural killer cell (NK) activity, decreased interleukin-2 (IL-2) production, and decreased serum thymulin activity in zinc deficient human subjects, which are reversible with zinc supplements. Several studies have shown that several micronutrients, including zinc, play a regulatory role in immune function (27).

Taste disorder

Altered taste sensation is comon in older people (15). Several investigators have studied the effect of zinc supplement in patients with hypogeusia. Yashide et al. (31) in a double blind trial studied 98 patients with taste disorder. Subjects were divided into four groups: zinc deficient, idiopathic, drug induced or other. Half of the subjects in each group received zinc gluconate (elemental zinc = 22.6 mg) three times a day for 4 months. Eighty two percent of the subjects in the treatment group vs 54 % subjects in the pacebo group reported improvement in symptoms. Most studies suggest that an elemental zinc supplement in a daily dosage of 25–100 mg may be effective for the treatment of dysgeusia and hypogeusia in zinc deficient patients.

Cardiovascular mortality

Several investigators have studied the role of trace elements, copper, and zinc in cardiovascular mortality. Reunanen et al. (25) studied the relationship between cardiovascular mortality and serum calcium, magnesium, copper, and zinc levels. The authors studied 230 men dying from cardiovascular diseases and 298 age-matched controls. They concluded that high serum copper and low serum zinc levels were associated with increased cardiovascular mortality. Hiller et al. (16) studied the serum zinc and serum lipid profiles in 778 subjects aged 22–80 years. The authors found that higher serum zinc levels, most notably those above the highest quintile, were associated with higher levels of total serum cholesterol, low density lipoproteins cholesterol, and triglycerides. No significant trend was noted for high density lipoprotein cholesterol.

Alzheimer's disease

Some investigators have shown that the patients with Alzheimer's disease have reduced zinc levels in the blood and brain tissue (29). The zinc levels have been found to be particularly low in the hippocampus in patients with Alzheimer's disease. Some investigators have suggested that zinc may regulate synaptic trans-mission in the hippocampus and, therefore, may play a significant role in the processing of memory. Constantindis (10), hypothesized that zinc deficiency in the hipocampus may contribute to the pathogenesis of neurofibullary . Tully et al. (29) studied the relationship between serum zinc level and neurofibrillary tangles in 12 elderly women with Alzheimer's disease. They found a moderate to strong negative correlation between serum zinc level drawn 12 months before death and neuro-fibrillary tangles.

Table 1. Daily zinc intake of healthy older people

Reference	Sample Size (n)	Zinc intake (mg) (mean ± SD)
Bunker et al. (1984) Am J Clin Nutr 40: 1096–1102	24	9.0 ± 2.6
Bunker et al. (1989) Age and Aging 18: 422–429	23	9.0
Swanson et al. (1988) Am J Clin Nutr 48: 343–349	53	9.2 ± 0.6
Gibson et al. (1985) J Gastroenterol 40: 296–302	NA	7.6 ± 3.3
Abdulla et al. (1989) Biol Trace Elem Res 21: 173–178	NA	7.2 ± 2.7
Prasad et al. (1993) Nutrition 9: 218–224	180	9.06

Age related macular degeneration

Some investigators have proposed that diet may influence the development of age related macular degeneration by influencing defense against oxidative damage. Studies in animal models have shown that the retina is susceptible to oxidative damage and that the retinal damage can be modulated by the presence of anti-oxidants and zinc (18). The data, however, remain non conclusive.

Nutritional status of zinc in older people

Several investigators have reported that dietary zinc intake declines with advancing age (Table 1). Low zinc intake in older people is believed to be due to a decline in caloric intake. Table 1 summarizes daily zinc intake of healthy older people in some of the published reports. The mean zinc intake varied from 7.2 to 10 mg/d, much below the recommended daily allowance of 15 mg/d for men and 12 mg/d for women.

Several studies have shown a low serum and leukocyte zinc concentration in institutionalized older people. Monget et al. (20) studied 756 institutionalized older people in France and found 58 % of men and 45.7 % of women in the study had low serum zinc concentrations. In another study, Stafford et al. (28) examined the zinc status of elderly institutionalized patients and concluded that the mean serum and leukocyte zinc concentrations were significantly lower in the institutionalized patients as compared to the older people living in the community. Rudman et al. (26) studied the essential nutrient intake of eating-dependent residents in a 190 bed Veterans Affairs Nursing Home. The authors found that, in 88 % of the eating dependent residents (EDR), the dietary intakes of three or more essential nutrients were below 50 % of the RDA. Most fequent and severely deficient were zinc, copper, and vitamin B6. A nutritional survey of 686 free living older people in the Boston area was conducted by the Human Nutrition Research Center on Aging at Tafts University, Boston, Massachusetts (14). The investigators found that zinc intake was below two thirds of the RDA in 50 % of the subjects studied. The investigators also found that the serum zinc levels declined with age and a negative relationship was found with the laxative use (30).

Intervention studies with zinc supplements

In this section some of the published intervention studies using zinc supplement will be reviewed.

Giroden et al. (12) examined the impact of a trace element and vitamin supplement on the incidence of infections in 81 older people living in a long-term care institution over a two year period. The subjects were randomly assigned to one of four treatment groups and received daily: (1) placebo, (2) trace elements (zinc 20 mg, selenium 100 ug), (3) vitamins (vitamin C 120 mg, β carotene 6 ug, ∝-tocopherol 15 mg) or (4) trace elements plus vitamins. The investigators recorded incidence of symptomatic respiratory and urogenital infections and mortality as the clinical outcomes. At the end of two year study period, the mortality was found to be similar among the four study groups. A significant decline (P < 0.01) in the mean number of infectious events was found in the group of subjects taking the trace elements. Compared with the placebo group, the subjects on trace elements had two to four times fewer infections during the two year study period.

Chandra (5) conducted a one year randomized double-blind placebo controlled trial in 96 men and women, 65 years and older, living independently in the community. The author tested the hypothesis that an optimum intake of all essential micronutrients in physiological amounts will result in an improvement in immune responses and reduce the frequency of infections in old age. The investigator found that several immunological responses were significantly improved in the supplemented group vs the placebo including the number of T cells, NK cells, lymphocyte response to phytohemaglutinin, IL-2 production, IL-2 receptor release, NK cell activity, and antibody response to influenza vaccine. Improvement in immunological responses was greater among subjects who at baseline had evidence of nutrient deficiency which was corrected after 12 months of supplement use.

Pike and Chandra (24) in a double-blind, placebo-controlled study examined the effect of a mineral and vitamin supplement on immune responses of 47 healthy, non-institutionalized older people aged 61–79 years. The number of CD3 T cells decreased significantly (P = 0.036) over the course of 12 months in the placebo group. This was associated with a decline in the CD4 helper T cells population and CD 4 to CD8 ration (P = 0.017). There was no significant decline in these cell counts in the supplemented group over the 12 month period. The number of CD 57 natural killer cells increased over one year in the supplemented group (P = 0.033). The CD 57 cells were significantly higher in the supplemented group vs the placebo group at 6 months (P = 0..036) and at 12 months (P = 0.012).

Chavance et al. (7) studied 218 subjects 60 years and older for 4 months and found no difference in the incidence of infections between the placebo group vs the group which received micronutrient supplements. In this study, the authors used a questionnaire to assess the incidence of infections. This is in contrast to the study by Chandra (5) where clinicians assessed subjects for infection and the duration of the study was one year. These differences in the methods may account for the differences in the outcome of the two studies (24).

Boukaiba et al. (4) studied 44 institutionalized subjects in a 16 week crossover study design to determine the effects of low dose zinc supplement (zinc gluconate 20 mg/d) on food intake, anthropometry, biochemical, and immunological indices. In the supplemented group, investigators found a partial but significant restoration of serum thymulin activity, improvement in food intake, serum albumin and thransthyretin concentrations, and a decline in serum copper concentration.

Fortes et al. (11) studied the effect of zinc and vitamin A supplementation on immune response in older people. In the zinc supplemented group, the authors found a significant increase in the number of CD4+, DR+, and T cells (P = 0.016) and cytotoxic T-lymphocytes (P = 0.005) whereas subjects who received vitamin A supplement had a reduction in the number of CD3+ T cells (P= 0.012) and CD4+ T cells (P = 0.012). This study showed that zinc supplementation improved cell medicated immunity whereas vitamin A supplementation had a deleterious effect on immune response in the study group.

At least two pulished reports have shown an adverse effect on the immune system of older adults with high dose zinc supplementation (100-150 mg/d) (3, 6).

Conclusion

The review of literature suggests that zinc deficiency is common in older people living independently in the community as well as those living in an institutionalized setting. Zinc is an essential nutrient and seems to play a significant role at various levels. Zinc seems to have an important effect on immune system. Some studies suggest that zinc supplementation, especially in older people with reduced zinc intake and lower serum zinc level, may favorably influence the immune system. On the other hand, excessive amounts of zinc supplement seem to have deleterious effects on the immune system. Micronutrient supplementation may be beneficial for older people at risk of malnutrition. More research, however, is needed to study the pathophysiologic effects of zinc in our body and zinc supplementation.

References

1. Abbasi AA, Rudman D (1994) Undernutrition in the nursing home: prevalence, consequences, causes and prevention. Nutr Rev 52 (4): 113–122
2. Agren MS (1990) Studies on zinc in wound healing. Acta Derm Venerol (Suppl) 154: 1–36
3. Bogden JD, Bendich A, Kemp FW, Bruening KS, Skurnick JH et al. (1994) Daily micronutrient supplements enhance delayed-type hypersensitivity skin test responses in older people. Am J Clin Nutr 60 (3): 437–447
4. Boukaiba N, Flament C, Acher S, Chappuis P, Piau A et al. (1993) A physiological amount of zinc supplementation: effects on nutritional, lipid, and thymic status in an elderly population. Am J Clin Nutr 57 (4): 566–572
5. Chandra RK (1992) Effect of vitamin and trace-element supplementation on immune responses and infection in elderly subjects. Lancet 340: 1124–1137
6. Chandra RK (1984) Excessive intake of zinc impairs immune response. JAMA 252: 1443–1446
7. Chavance M, Herbeth B, Lemoine A, Zhu BP (1993) Does multivitamin supplementation prevent infections in healthy elderly subjects? A controlled Trial. Internat J Vitam Nutr Res 63: 11–16
8. Clayton RJ (1972) A double-blind trial of oral zinc sulfate in patitnets with leg ulcers. J Clin Pract 26: 368–370
9. Dachowski EJ, Plummer VA, Greaves VM (1975) Venous leg ulceration: skin oil serum zinc concentrations. Acta Derm Venerol 55: 497–498
10. Constantinidis J (1991) The hypothesis of zinc deficiency in the pathogenesis of neurofibrillary tangles. Med Hypoth 35: 319–323

11. Fortes C, Forastiere F, Agabiti N, Fano V, Pacifici R, Virgili F, Piras G et al. (1998) The effect of zinc and vitamin A supplementation on immune response in an older population. J Am Geriatr Soc 46: 19–26

12. Girodon F, Lombard M, Golan P, Brunet-Leconte P, Monget A, Arnaud J et al. (1997) Effect of micronutrient supplementation on infection in institutionalized elderly subjects: A controlled trial. Ann Nutr Metab 41: 98–107

13. Hallbook T, Lanner E (1972) Serum zinc and healing of venous leg ulcers. Lancet ii: 780–782

14. Hartz SC, Russell RM, Rosenberg IH (eds) (1990) Nutrition in the Elderly: The Boston Nutritional Status Survey. London: Smith-Gordon

15. Heyneman CA (1996) Zinc deficiency and taste disorders. The annals of Pharmacotherapy 30: 186–187

16. Hiller R, Seigel D, Sperduto D, Blair N, Burton T (1995) Serum zinc and serum lipid profiles in 778 adults. Ann Epidemiol 5: 490–496

17. Krasinski SD, Russell RM, Samloft JM, Jacob RA et al. (1986) Fundic atrophic gastritis in an elderly population: effect on hemoglobin and several serum nutritional indicators. J Am Geriatr Soc 34: 800–806

18. Mares-Perlman JA, Klein R, Klein B, Greger JL, Brady WE, Palta M, Ritter LL (1996) Association of zinc and antioxidant nutrients with age related maculopathy. Arch Ophthalmol 114: 991–997

19. Mobarhan S, Trumbore LS (1992) Nutritional problems of the elderly. Clinics in Geriatr Med 7 (2): 191–214

20. Monget AL, Galan P, Presiosi P, Keller H, Bourgeois C et al. (1996) Micronutrient status in elderly people. Internat J Vit Nutr Res 66: 71–76

21. Niedner R, Wokalek H, Schopf E (1986) Influence of zinc on the healing of wounds. Z Hautkr 61: 741–742

22. Norman JN, Rahmat A, Smith G (1975) Effects of supplements of zinc salts on the healing of granulating wounds in the rat and guinea pig. J Nutr 105: 815–821

23. Phillips A, Davidson M, Greaves MW (1977) Venous leg ulceration: evaluation of zinc treatment, serum zinc and rate of healing. Clin Exp Dermatol 2: 395–399

24. Pike J, Chandra RK (1995) Effect of vitamin and trace element supplementation on immune indices in healthy elderly. Internat J Vit Nutr Res 65: 117–120

25. Reunanen A, Knekt P, Marniemi J, Maki J, Maatela J, Aromaa A (1996) Serum calcium, magnesium, copper, and zinc and risk of cardiovascular death. European J of Clin Nutr 50: 431–437

26. Rudman D, Abbasi AA, Isaacson K, Karpuik E (1995) Observations on the nutrient intakes of eating dependent nursing home residents: underutilization of micronutrient supplements. J Am Coll Nutr 14 (6): 604–613

27. Santos-Neto L, Tosta CE, Dorea JG (1992) Zinc reverses the increased sensitivity of lymphocytes from aged subjects to the antiproliferative effect of prostaglandin E2. Clinical Immunology, Immunopathology 64 (3): 184–187

28. Stafford W, Smith RG, Lewis SJ, Henery E, Stephen PJ et al. (1998) A Study of zinc status of elderly institutionalized patients. Age & Ageing 17: 42–48

29. Tully CL, Snowdon DA, Markesbery WR (1995) Serum zinc, senile plaques, and neurofibrillary tangles: findings from the nun study. Neuroloreport 6: 2105–2108

30. Wood R (1990) Zinc. In: Hartz SC, Russell RM, Rosenberg IH (eds) Nutrition in the Elderly: The Boston Nutritional Status Survey. London: Smith-Gordon

31. Yoshida S, Endo S, Tomita H (1991) A double-blind study of the therapeutic efficacy of zinc gluconate on taste disorder. Auris-Nasus Larynx 18: 153–161

Author's address:

Adil Abbasi, MD
22095 Peterhill Ct.
Waukesha, WI 53186, USA

Preventive nutrition services for aging populations

B. E. Millen

Associate Dean for Research, Boston University School of Public Health, Boston, MA, USA

Population aging is a global phenomenon (9, 20, 37, 38, 51). In the last 40 years, average life expectancy worldwide increased from 46 years to 65 years and the gap in life expectancy between all countries narrowed from 25 years to 13.3 years (20). These demographic transitions have brought about dramatic changes in the world's health needs. Chronic diseases, such as heart disease, hypertension and stroke, diabetes, pulmonary disease, and certain cancers are either rapidly emerging or are already established at high rates globally (41). Chronic diseases of aging account for nearly half of population morbidity and mortality in the developing regions of the world and over 85 % of deaths and disability in developed regions (9, 20, 37, 38, 41). Of particular importance to this discussion is that malnutrition, which in this context includes both nutritional excesses and deficiencies, is one of the few preventable risk factors for chronic diseases (41). Carefully planned population-based nutrition interventions can lower risk for chronic diseases and their adverse outcomes. High-risk nutrition interventions can also be used to reach particularly vulnerable segments of the population, such as extremely frail elders, to reduce the prevalence of nutrient deficiencies. Clearly, the prevention of nutrition-related problems in the population, including older persons, has important global health implications.

The purpose of this chapter is to examine the determinants of nutritional risk in elders and to explore opportunities for preventive nutrition services in older populations. U.S. policy statements and mechanisms for the promotion of nutritional well-being in elder populations are emphasized. A global initiative, called InterHealth, that is sponsored by the World Health Organization and aimed at lowering chronic disease risk in aging populations is also highlighted (37, 38).

Nutrition and physical health promotion in advancing age

Nutritional well-being is essential for the promotion and maintenance of the health, independence, and quality of life of older individuals (10, 16, 55, 58). In addition to mitigating health problems, proper nutrition improves the management of many chronic diseases, and extend years of healthy living with advancing age (59). Conversely, the presence of malnutrition is a primary risk factor for recurrent hospitalizations and costly, extended institutionalization, comorbidity, surgical complications, and delayed recuperation from physical injury and trauma (45).

While American elders are relatively healthy, over 85 % of free-living persons who are 65 years and older have one or more chronic health problems that could be improved with proper nutrition and many suffer from various forms of malnutrition (16, 55)

The myriad nutritional problems of the older population span a broad spectrum ranging from frank nutrient deficiencies, such as protein-energy malnutrition, to evidence of nutritional excesses, including obesity, dyslipidemia, hypertension, and higher than recommended levels of dietary lipids and other nutrients (7, 11, 12, 15, 25, 55, 57, 58). Nutrient deficiencies are relatively uncommon in the free-living elder population; up to 15 % of elders are affected. Nonetheless, up to 40 % of the frail, homebound elderly and a similar proportion of the institutionalized older population may suffer from protein-energy malnutrition and frank nutrient deficiencies (such as folate or vitamin B12 deficiency) (55). Dietary imbalances are more common. In national nutrition studies, low dietary intakes of energy, fiber, calcium, magnesium, antioxidants, certain B vitamins, and other micronutrients are common in older persons (14, 26, 52, 69). As many as one in four older people may consume low levels of nutrients which results in increased risk for nutrient deficiencies. These micronutrient imbalances may also increase risks for certain nutrition-related chronic diseases, such as diabetes and heart disease, and their complications (26, 55, 60).

Risk factors for nutrient deficiencies in the older U.S. population are not well understood. Low nutrient intake is associated with low nutrient intake are acute and chronic medical problems, particularly the presence of multiple, coexisting health problems; polypharmacy; losses of functional capacity; advanced age; poor oral health; loss of appetite; altered taste and olfactory acuity; social isolation; depression and other psychological disturbances; poverty; lack of nutrition knowledge; and susceptibility to fraud (3, 13, 17, 52, 60, 70, 76, 81). Among the non-institutionalized elderly, those who are homebound and frail appear to be particularly at risk for nutrient deficiencies (39, 60, 81). In addition, poverty and minority ethnicity increase levels of food insecurity, limit access to food and nutrition services, and increase risks for malnutrition in elder populations (67).

In contrast to nutrient deficiency syndromes, nutritional excesses, including obesity, appear to be quite common in the older American population. It is estimated that 40 % of older persons are overweight or obese by accepted clinical standards (2, 39, 81). Up to half of the free-living U.S. population 60 years of age and older consume diets with higher than recommended levels of nutrients, such as fat and sodium, which may have detrimental impacts on health (2, 39, 55, 67). Nutritional excesses impose increased risk not only for the development of chronic diseases such as hypertension, coronary heart disease, diabetes, and certain forms of cancer, but also for their adverse complications and outcomes including death and physical disabilities (39, 54).

Little research has characterized the determinants of dietary excesses and related health problems in the older population. One recent study in a population-based sample of free-living elders in New England (59) suggested that smoking and male gender were associated with nutritional excesses, such as higher than recommended levels of nutrients (particularly dietary lipids). Those elders who continued to smoke were more apt to consume high dietary lipid intake. Older women, compared with elder men, were more likely to comply with recent recommendations for "heart healthy" nutrient intake (59).

There are significant gaps exist in our understanding of nutrition-related problems and their etiology in the elder population. Indeed, Horwath (21) recently reviewed over 90 studies on diet and nutritional status of older individuals and concluded that the majority were conducted in small, highly selected samples with limited generalizability. As a consequence, priority research areas have been identified investigation: the prevalence of nutrition-related problems and their etiology in various segments of the older population including the frail, homebound elderly; the role of nutritional factors in the etiology and prevention of chronic diseases and in age-related impairments in organ system function; nutrition interventions that are consistent with relieving common causes of morbidity in older adults; relationships between nutrition, physical functioning, and health; and the nutritional determinants of cognitive and physical functioning and quality of life in advanced age (26, 44, 66, 72, 81).

US national public nutrition policies and recommendations

In the last several decades, growing concern over nutritional risk in the older population has led to the development of key public policy statements to improve the nutritional status of older Americans and to enhance the delivery of nutrition and related health services. The most recent US policy directive, Healthy People 2000 (73), is consistent with other national recommendations including the Office of the Surgeon General (66,72), the Institute of Medicine (26), and the Committee on Diet and Health of the National Research Council (44). The Year 2000 report placed particular emphasis on the following goals: reducing the morbidity and mortality associated with chronic diseases including heart disease, hypertension and stroke, certain cancers, diabetes, and osteoporosis; increasing years of healthy and independent living; increasing abilities to perform activities of daily living, including shopping for food and preparing meals; improving access to and use of supportive social and primary health care services; and improving behavioral risk profiles (diet; alcohol and tobacco use; and physical activity). Specific nutrition-related objectives for older persons placed attention on reducing total and saturated fat and sodium intakes; assuring adequate dietary levels of essential micronutrients; reducing the prevalence of obesity; improving access to food and nutrition services (particularly home-delivered meals and congregate feeding); and promoting the availability of nutrition services, in particular, nutritional assessment, counseling and education, provided by qualified nutrition professionals to older individuals (73). These recommendations also agree closely with the following reports: the Food Guide Pyramid and related Dietary Guidelines (68), the general adult population recommendations set forth by the Committee on Diet and Health (44), the National Cholesterol Education Program (13), and the National Cancer Institute (19).

In addition to these policy directives, the Food and Nutrition Board of the (US) National Academy of Sciences (84) has published guidelines, termed the Dietary Reference Intakes (DRIs), which expand and replace the Recommended Dietary

Allowances (RDAs). They are designed to provide quantitative estimates of nutrient intake to assure the adequacy of intakes for energy, macronutrients, and selected micronutrients. They can be used for many purposes, such as diet and menu planning, in community and institutional settings for health services delivery. The DRIs set nutrient intake guidelines for two older adult age groups, those 51–70 years of age and those over age 70.

Additional recommendations set forth by the Nutrition Screening Initiative (NSI) deserve particular attention (18, 34, 44, 45, 48, 49, 77–80). While not a governmental body, NSI is a collaboration of over 25 professional organizations in the United States that are interested in improving the nutrition and health status of the older population. The initiative is committed to increasing public awareness of the nutritional needs of the older population, promoting optimal nutrition in advancing age, and developing strategies for nutritional risk assessment and intervention planning. Through a consensus-building process and ongoing research, the Nutrition Screening Initiative has developed methods for increasing consumer awareness of nutrition problems and methods for the in-depth detection of nutritional risk among older people (18, 19, 34, 44, 45, 48, 49, 78–80).

The NSI has also developed guidelines and recommends methods for screening and in-depth evaluation of nutritional risk in older populations and the designation of appropriate interventions (48, 49). The methods include a validated, self-administered 10 item checklist for assessing warning signs of poor nutritional status in older adults (80). The NSI has urged clinicians to incorporate nutritional screening as part of routine activities in free-living and institutionalized elderly populations in order to develop appropriate interventions. Several recent publications provide guidelines for professionals who are involved in nutritional care of older individuals (44, 45, 48, 49).

Most recently, the NSI published dietary management guidelines for chronic disease care in older individuals (77). The publication relies on evidence-based information, where available to develop specific recommended strategies for managing the clinical features of various health conditions including: cancer, chronic obstructive pulmonary disease, congestive heart failure, coronary heart disease, dementia, diabetes mellitus, hypertension, failure to thrive, osteoporosis, and pneumonia. Consensus-based information was used to develop recommendations for dietary intervention where research was more limited or unavailable. Information was also assessed and provided on the expected outcomes of nutrition intervention and the profile of suitable providers of professional nutrition care. The report highlights the results of several recent research investigations on the cost-effectiveness of nutrition care in older adults in hospital and community settings. It was estimated that the delivery of appropriate nutrition intervention to elders would save up to $ 1.3 billion in health-related costs by the year 2002 (77, p. 1).

In summary, there is striking consensus in recent national policy statements and the recommendations of professional groups that nutritional risk assessment and interventions are important components of health care delivery to older persons. There is recognition that the nutritional problems of the elderly span a spectrum from frank nutrient deficiencies, like protein-energy malnutrition, to nutritional excesses, exhibited in obesity, hypercholesterolemia, hypertension, and diabetes. There is also attention given to the importance of assuring that an individual's dietary intake is adequate to meet nutrient requirements, particularly among those who may experience food insecurity for financial, cognitive, functional or other reasons. These recommendations stress that preventive nutrition is as important among elders as in younger populations. Dietary management for the prevention of the chronic diseases of aging and their adverse complications are likewise evident. Guidelines emphasize the balancing of energy intake to maintain ideal body weight, lower total and saturated fat intake, reduced sodium and sugar intake, and increased fiber-, calcium-, and fluoride-containing foods. The integration of community-based services for elderly among the multidisciplinary array of service providers and agencies is also considered of paramount importance.

The following section examines the available US frameworks for the delivery of community-based preventive nutrition programs and services to elders, in particularly the Elder Nutrition Program (53, 67). A smaller initiative, the Food Stamp program which provides food coupons and income supplements to poor elders is discussed elsewhere (1, 5, 75). A discussion of Medicare and Medicaid, the primary US mechanisms for the financing of preventive and therapeutic nutrition services for older persons in US health care delivery settings is beyond our scope but is summarized in a recent report (35, 71).

Community-based preventive nutrition services for older americans

Title III and VI elder nutrition program

The largest publicly-funded and longest standing program of coordinated com-munity- and home-based preventive health-related and social services for older Americans is the Elder Nutrition Program (ENP) (39, 58, 67). ENP was established by the Older Americans Act of 1972; it distributes funding to the US states (through State Units on Aging (SUAs)), United States territories, and Indian Tribal Organi-zations (ITOs) for a national network of programs that provide congregate and home-delivered meals for elderly people. This program was designed to reduce risks for food insecurity and nutrient deficiencies as well as social isolation in elder Americans, particularly the poor and minority elderly. ENP funding helps main-tain an elaborate infrastructure of Area Agencies on Aging (AoA) and Nutrition Projects at the regional and local levels, respectively, for the delivery of nutrition and related health and supportive social services to older clients. AoA currently dis-tributes about $ 500 million annually in ENP federal funding to a national network of 57 State and Territorial Units on Aging, 670 Area Agencies on Aging, and over 200 Indian Tribal organizations (ITOs). It is estimated that ENP provides services to 2.3 million elders through community sites and delivered meals and other in-home services to over 877,000 frail elders (53, 67).

ENP sites are required to provide at least one meal a day that meets one-third of the recommended dietary allowances (RDA) and to operate 5 or more days a week (67). Lessor known but of great importance is the role of ENP in administering and/or delivering other health and supportive social services including: access initiatives (transportation, outreach, information, and referral), in-home services (homemaker, home health aide, personal care, and chore assistance), and community-based health and supportive social activities (medical screening, case management, legal and financial assistance and counseling, physical fitness programs, rehabilitation services, and social and recreational activities (53, 67).

ENP maintains two major meal service delivery systems – one which provides community-based, congregate (group) and individual services to the ambulatory older population and the other which delivers services to the frail, homebound elderly. ENP services emphasize preventive nutrition, particularly the provision of congregate and home-delivered meals (often called meals on wheels), as well as nutrition screening, education, and counseling.

Federal law mandates that ENP be available to all older Americans (those 60 years and older and their spouses regardless of age) and that client contributions (payment) for services be strictly voluntary. Within federal funding limitations, the ENP attempts to strategically place local projects in community facilities that serve those in greatest need – the poor, minority, and frail elderly. Older individuals voluntarily become ENP clients and are referred by health and medical providers (such as hospitals, private physicians, group medical practices, social service agencies, etc.) as well as informal family and social networks.

Many researchers have attempted to determine the impact of ENP on the nutritional well-being and health of older participants (6, 28, 29, 33, 45, 85) From these reports, it appears that ENP attracts "high risk" elders, improves food and nutrient intake among participants, and provides beneficial socialization and recreation. Balsam and Rogers (4) found that many NPOA sites were compelled to become innovative in meeting the nutritional needs of its participants. Beyond the congregate and home meals that are required by law, these researchers found that many nutrition programs across the nation provide therapeutic diets; food pantries; ethnic meals; luncheon clubs; breakfast, weekend, and evening meals; and meals for the homeless older population.

A recent comprehensive evaluation of ENP (36, 53) further informed national health policy development. The national evaluation found that ENP clients had profiles associated with considerably higher risk for nutrition problems including that they have on average 2–3 coexisting chronic diseases, various degrees of limitation in functional capacity, and high rates of hospitalization and short-term institutionalization. Clients were older by 4–6 years than US elders overall and included proportionately more females and minority individuals. There are more than twice the proportion of impoverished elders being served by Title III than are in the general population. The proportion of low-income minority elders that receive Title III services is about four times greater than their proportion in the overall older population.

Results of the evaluation indicated that the program made significant improvements in participants' levels of nutrient intake and patterns of socialization. The mean daily nutrient intake of ENP clients approached or exceeded the guidelines for nutrient intake for most nutrients studied. In addition, clients had favorable intakes of dietary fat and cholesterol. The ENP meals were also found to contribute between 30 and 50 % of total daily nutrient intake among congregate and homebound program participants (53, 85). Socialization was also a key research outcome. Results of the ENP evaluation indicate that ENP clients experienced a 17 % increase in monthly social contacts (53, 85). The importance of maintaining nutritional well-being in older persons has been demonstrated in other research (24, 32, 40, 65, 66). The relationship between socialization and reduced mortality among elders has also been confirmed in longitudinal research studies (22, 27, 61, 63, 83).

A number of European countries, including England, Sweden, Denmark, the Netherlands, and Great Britain, have also devised or are also testing new strategies for the delivery of community-based and in-home long-term care services (8). These efforts have arisen over the past decade in response to the progressive aging of European populations and concerns over the rising national investments in acute and long-term institutional care. While none of the existing international models have central focus in nutrition, like ENP, all appear to include congregate meals or "meal-on-wheels" as essential components of care. One model that is quite similar to ENP (72) has developed local community centers to manage a wide range of referral services for homebound and ambulatory elders and to provide congregate or in-home meals and social, educational, and recreational activities. Common features of the various European models are increased emphasis on decentralization of financing and coordination of health and related services at the local community level; greater acknowledgment of the importance of informal care activities (from family members, etc.); expansion of provider networks beyond those that are publicly-funded to include voluntary and private sectors; and closer matching of patient needs with a varying, versus fixed, set of services (8). Ongoing research suggests that configurations of health and related services in these ways may improve the quality of care and service delivery efficiency, and control or lower institutional health care costs (8, 31).

Recognizing the serious tolls associated with the chronic diseases of aging, the World Health Organization introduced the InterHealth Programme, a collaboration of nation's in all regions of the world (37, 38). The purpose of this global initiative is to reduce risks for chronic diseases at the population level through integrated policy directives and behavioral interventions. A central features in their integrated risk factor modification strategies is the promotion of sound eating practices in the population. InterHealth recognizes that poor nutrition is associated with increased risks for multiple chronic diseases, including coronary heart disease, hypertension, diabetes mellitus, certain forms of cancer, and osteoporosis. Countries participating in InterHealth have established national policy statements on nutrition for non-communicable disease (NCD) prevention and control and have also established models for nutrition intervention at the national, community, household, and individual levels. InterHealth has also provided a mechanism for the systematic evaluation of its community-based interventions and the global sharing of information on strategies for chronic disease risk reduction in populations throughout the developed and developing world (16). Further details are beyond the scope of this discussion, but the InterHealth Nutrition Initiative has been recently reviewed (37, 38).

Conclusion

The health and nutrition status of older people has improved in this century, but many continue to have unmet needs for nutritional services. The most prevalent nutritional problems of people aged 65 years and older in the US appear to be the nutrition-related chronic diseases of aging, including coronary heart disease, hypertension, diabetes, cancer, and osteoporosis. These affect many, if not most older people. There are also distinct groups of elders, notably those who are socially isolated, very old and frail, poor, and of minority populations, who are at greatest risk for nutrient deficiencies. The factors and personal characteristics that place the older population at risk of nutrition problems are poorly understood. Considerable future research, of both a basic and applied nature, is needed to resolve these information deficits and to provide the critical basis for advocacy on behalf of elders and their nutritional needs.

The Elder Nutrition Program provides a framework in the US for the delivery of nutrition and related health and supportive social services to elders. The recent national evaluation provides strong evidence of its success and favorable impacts on nutrition and socialization of elder participants. There is also emerging evidence that the agencies involved in the delivery of ENP have evolved into an infrastructure that is increasingly involved in the integration and coordination of services in order to establish a continuum of health related services, beyond simply meals, that support the independent living of older clients.

Models for community-based preventive nutrition services and programs for aging populations are also emerging internationally. Such initiatives generally consider the delivery of congregate and home meals. Many also consider the integration of supportive social services that can aid in maintaining independent living among elders. The World Health Organization has also established the Inter-Health Initiative to promote the reduction in chronic diseases in aging populations. This program is a model of global collaboration on effort is a model for population-based preventive intervention planning.

Further advances in life expectancy and the quality of life of older populations throughout the world will depend on continued improvements in health, the prevention and early treatment of diseases or their complications, and better understanding of the aging process. Nutritional interventions and related services will play a central role in the promotion of successful aging.

References

1. Akin JS, Guilkey DK, Popkin BM et al. (1985) The impact of federal transfer programs on the nutrient intake of elderly individuals. J Hum Resources 20: 382–404
2. Assistant Secretary for Aging. Food and Nutrition for Life: Malnutrition and Older Americans. Washington, DC: Administration on Aging, DHHS, Dec. 1994
3. Bailey LB (1980) Vitamin B$_{12}$ status of elderly persons from urban low-income households. J Am Geriatr Soc 28: 276–78
4. Balsam AL, Rogers BL (1988) Service innovations in the ederly nutrition program: Strategies for meeting unmet needs. Boston, MA. Tufts University School of Nutrition

5. Butler JS, Ohls JC, Posner BM (1985) The effect of the food stamp program on the nutrient intake of the eligible elderly. J Hum Resources 20: 405–19

6. Caliendo MA, Smith J (1981) Factors influencing the nutrition knowledge and dietary intake of participants in the Title III-c meal program. J Nutr Elderly 1: 65–77

7. Carroll MD, Abraham S, Dresser CM (eds) (1983) Dietary Intake Source Data: U.S., 1976–80, NHANES I, II. Hyattsville, MD: National Center for Health Statistics

8. Coleman BJ (1995) European models of long-term care in the home and community. Int J Hlth Serv 25: 455–74

9. Diet, Nutrition and the Prevention of Chronic Disease (1990) Report of a WHO Study Group. Technical report series 797. Geneva: World Health Organization

10. Dwyer JT (1991) Screening Older Americans' Nutritional Health: Current Practices and Future Possibilities. Washington, DC: The Nutrition Screening Initiative

11. Dwyer JT (1993) Nutrition concerns and problems of the aged. In: Satin D (ed) Clinical Care of the Aged Person. New York: Oxford University Press

12. Dwyer JT, Coletti J, Campbell D (1991) Maximizing nutrition in the second fifty. Clin Appl Nutr 4: 19–31

13. Expert Panel on Detection, Evaluation and Treatment of High Blood Cholesterol in Adults (1993) Summary of the Second Report of the National Cholesterol Education Program (NCEP) Expert Panel on Detection, Evaluation and Treatment of High Blood Cholesterol in Adults (Adult Treatment Panel II). JAMA 269, 3015–23

14. Food Research and Action Center (1987) A National Survey of Nutritional Risk Among the Elderly. Washington, DC: Food Research and Action Center

15. Goodwin JS (1989) Social, psychological and physical factors affecting the nutritional status of elderly subjects: Separating cause and effect. Am J Clin Nutr 50: 1201–09

16. Guidelines for Protocols for Local Demonstration Projects (1990) Division of Noncommunicable Diseases and Health Technology. INTERHEALTH. Geneva: World Health Organization

17. Guthrie HA, Black K, Madden JP (1972) Nutritional practices of elderly citizens in rural Pennsylvania. Gerontologist 12: 330–35

18. Ham RJ (1991) Indicators of Poor Nutritional Status in Older Americans. Washington, DC: Nutrition Screening Initiative

19. Havas S, Heimendinger J, Reynolds K, Baranowski T, Nicklas TA et al. (1994) 5 a day for better health: A new research initiative. J Am Diet Assoc 94: 32–36

20. Health for All in the 21st Century (1998) Geneva. World Health Organization

21. Horwath CC (1989) Dietary intake studies in elderly people. World Rev Nutr Diet 59: 1–70

22. House JS, Robbins C, Metzner HL (1982) The association of social relationships and activities with mortality: prospective evidence from the Tecumseh Community Health Study. Am J Epidemiol 116: 123–40

23. House Select Committee on Aging, Subcommittee on Health and Long-Term Care (1984) Quackery: A $10 Billion Scandal. Washington, DC: US Government Printing Office; Publication No. 98–435

24. Hubert HB, Bloch DA, Fries JF (1993) Risk factors for disability in an aging cohort. The NHANES I Epidemiologic follow-up study. J Rheumatol 20: 480–88

25. Hutchinson M, Munro HN (1986) Nutrition and Aging. New York, NY: Academic Press

26. Institute of Medicine, Division of Health Promotion and Disease Prevention (1992) The Second Fifty Years. Promoting Health and Preventing Disability. Berg RL, Cassells JS (eds) Washington, DC: National Academy Press

27. Kaplan GA, Salomen JT, Cohen RD, , Brand RJ, Syme SL, Puska P (1988) Social connections and mortality from all causes fand from cardiovascular disease: prospective evidence from eastern Finland. Am J Epidemiol 128: 370–80

28. Kirschner Associates Inc. & Opinion Research Corporation (1980) Longitudinal Evaluation of the National Washington, DC: Administration on Aging; US Department of Health, Education, and Welfare Publ. no. 80–20249

29. Kohrs MB (1980) Association of participation in a nutritional program for the elderly with nutritional status. Am J Clin Nutr 33: 2643–56

30. Kohrs MB, O'Hanlon P, Eklund D (1978) Title VII nutrition program for the elderly, I: contribution to one day's dietary intake. J Am Diet Assoc 72: 487–92
31. Kristiansen R (1992) Elderly people in a large Danish city. Dan Med Bull 39: 234–36
32. La Croix AZ, Guralnick JM, Berkman LF, Wallace RB, Satterfield S (1993) Maintaining mobility in later life. Am J Epidemiol 137: 858–69
33. LeClerc H, Thornbury ME (1983) Dietary intakes of Title III meal program recipients and non-recipients. J Am Diet Assoc 83: 573–77
34. Lipschitz DA (1991) The Development of an Approach to Nutrition Screening for Older Americans. Washington, DC: Nutrition Screening Initiative.
35. The Medicare Program and Nutrition Services (1998) June 1997. Http://www.eatright. org.med. html. The American Dietetic Association
36. Millen BE, Levine E: A Continuum of Nutrition Services for Older Americans. In: Chernoff R (ed) Geriatric Nutrition. The Health Professional's Handbook. Gaithersburg, Md. In press
37. Millen Posner B, Franz M, Quatromoni P, InterHealth Steering Committee (1994) Nutrition and the global risk for chronic diseases: The InterHealth nutrition initiative. Nutr Rev 52: 201–7
38. Millen Posner B, Quatromoni PA, Franz M (1994) Nutrition policies and intervention for chronic disease risk reduction in international settings: The InterHealth nutrition initiative. Nutr Rev 52: 179–87
39. Millen BM, Saffel-Shrier S, Dwyer J, Franz MM (1993) Position of the American Dietetic Association: Nutrition, aging, and the continuum of health care. J Am Diet Assoc 93: 80–82
40. Murphy SP, Davis MA, Neuhaus JM, Lein D (1990) Factors influencing dietary adequacy and energy intake in older Americans. J Nutr Ed 22: 284–91
41. Murray CJL, Lopez AD (1996) The Global Burden of Disease. Geneva. World Health Organization
42. National Center for Health Statistics (1988) Health, United States-1987. US Dept of Health and Human Services publications PHS 88-1232. Washington, DC: US Government Printing Office
43. National Center for Health Statistics (1986) Aging in the Eighties: Preliminary Data from the Supplement on Aging to the National Health Interview Survey. Hyattsville, Md: National Center for Health Statistics. Advance Data from Vital and Health Statistics, N 115. US Dept of Health and Human Services publication PHS 86-1250
44. National Research Council (1989b) Diet and Health. Implications for Reducing Chronic Disease Risk. Washington, DC: National Academy Press
45. The Nutrition Screening Initiative (1994) Incorporating Nutrition Screening and Interventions into Medical Practice. A Monograph for Physicians. Washington, DC: The Nutrition Screening Initiative
46. The Nutrition Screening Initiative (1992) Nutrition Interventions Manual for Professionals Caring for Older Americans. Washington, DC: The Nutrition Screening Initiative
47. Nestle M, Lee PR, Fullarton JE (1983) Nutrition and the Elderly: A Working Paper for the Administration on Aging. Policy Paper No. 2. San Francisco, CA: Aging Health Policy Center, University of California
48. The Nutrition Screening Initiative (1991) Nutrition Screening Manual for Professionals Caring for Older Americans. Washington, DC: Nutrition Screening Initiative
49. The Nutrition Screening Initiative (1991) Report of Nutrition Screening 1: Toward a Common View. Washington, DC: Nutrition Screening Initiative
50. Orth-Gomer K, Johnson JV (1987) Social network interaction and mortality: A six year follow-up study of a random sample of the Swedish population. J Chron Dis 40: 949–57
51. Omran AR (1977) A century of epidemiologic transition in the United States. Prev Med 6: 30–51
52. Ponza M, Ohls JC, Millen BE (1996) Serving Elders at Risk. The Older Americans Act Nutrition Programs. National Evaluation of the Elderly Nutrition Program, 1993-1995. Washington, DC: US Department of Health and Human Services. Office of the Assistant Secretary for Aging. Office of the Assistant Secretary for Planning and Evaluation

53. Ponza M, Ohls JC & Posner BM. (1994). Elderly Nutrition Program Evaluation Literature Review. Princeton, NJ: MATHEMATICA Policy Research, Inc.
54. Posner BM (1979) Nutrition and the Elderly. Lexington, MA: Health & Co.
55. Posner BM, Fanelli MT, Krachenfels MM, Saffel-Schreier S (1987) Position of the American Dietetic Association: Nutrition, aging and the continuum of health care. J Am Diet Assoc 87: 344–47
56. Posner BM, Jette AM, Smith KW, Miller DR (1993a) Nutrition and health risks in the elderly: The Nutrition Screening Initiative. Am J Public Health 83: 972–78
57. Posner BM, Krachenfels MM (1987) Nutrition services in the continuum of care. Clin Geriatr Med 3: 261–74
58. Posner BM, Levine EL (1991) Nutrition services for older Americans. In: Geriatric Nutrition: A Health Professional's Handbook. Gaithersburg, MD: Aspen Publishers
59. Posner BM, Jette A, Smigelski C, Miller D, Mitchell P (1994) Nutritional Risk in New England Elders. J Gerontol Med Sci 49: M123–32
60. Posner BM, Smigelski CG, Krachenfels MM (1987) Dietary characteristics and nutrient intake in an urban homebound population. J Am Diet Assoc 87: 452–6
61. Seeman TE, Kaplan GA, Knudsen L, Cohen R, Guralnick J (1987) Social network ties and mortality among the elderly in the Alameda County study. Am J Epidemiol 126: 714–23
62. Shoenbach VJ, Kaplan BH, Fredman L, Kleinbaum DG (1986) Social ties and mortality in Evans County, Georgia. Am J Epidemiol 123: 577–91
63. Shye D, Mullooly JP, Freeborn DK, Pope CR (1995) Gender differences in the relationship between social network support and mortality: a longitudinal study of an elderly cohort. Soc Sci Med 41: 935–47
64. Sullivan DH, Walls RC, Bopp MM (1995) Protein-energy undernutrition and risk of mortality within one year of hospital discharge: A follow-up study. J Am Ger Soc 43: 506–12
65. Sullivan DH, Walls RC (1994) Impact of nutritional status on morbidity in a population of geriatric rehabilitation patients. J Am Ger Soc 42: 471–77
66. Surgeon General's Workshop on Health Promotion and Aging (1988) Washington, DC: US Government Printing Office; Publication No. 1988-201-875/83669
67. Torres-Gil FM, Lloyd JL, Carlin J (1995) Role of elderly nutrition in home and community-based care. Persp Appl Nutr 2: 9–15
68. US Department of Agriculture (1992) The Food Guide Pyramid. Home and Garden Bulletin No. 252. Hyattsville, MD: Human Nutrition Information Service
69. US Department of Health and Human Services & US Department of Agriculture (1986) Nutrition Monitoring in the U.S.: A Report from the Joint Nutrition Monitoring Evaluation Committee. Washington, DC: US Government Printing Office; US Public Health Service; USDHHS publ.PHS 86-1255
70. US Department of Health and Human Services (1972) Ten-State Nutrition Survey, V: Dietary. Atlanta, GA: Centers for Disease Control; US Dept of Health and Human Services Publ. no. HSM 72-8133
71. US Department of Health and Human Services (1997) Health Care Financing Administration. Your Medicare Handbook 1997. Washington DC. US Government Printing Office. 552–158
72. US Department of Health and Human Services Public Health Service (1988) Aging. In: The Surgeon General's Report on Nutrition and Health. Washington DC: US Government Printing Office; DHHS (PHS) Publication No. 88-50210
73. US Department of Health and Human Services. Public Health Service (1992) Healthy People 2000. National Health Promotion and Disease Prevention Objectives. Full Report, with Commentary. Boston, MA: Jones and Bartlett Publishers
74. US Senate Special Committee on Aging, the American Association of Retired Persons, the Federal Council on the Aging, & the US Administration on Aging (1991) Aging America. Trends and Projections. 1991 Edition. Washington, DC: US. Department of Health and Human Services; DHHS Publ. No. (FCoA) 91-28001)
75. US Senate Special Committee on Aging (1987) Developments in Aging: 1986. A Report of the Special Committee on Aging. Washington DC: US Government Printing Office ASI No. 25144.3

76. Vaughan LA, Manore MM (1988) Dietary patterns and nutritional status of low income, free-living elderly. Food Nutr News 60: 27–30
77. White JV (ed) The Role of Nutrition in Chronic Disease Care. Washington DC: The Nutrition Screening Initiative, 1997
78. White JV (1991) Risk Factors Associated with Poor Nutritional Status in Older Americans. Washington, DC: Nutrition Screening Initiative
79. White JV, Dwyer JT, Millen Posner B et al. (1992) Nutrition Screening Initiative: Development and Implementation of the Public Awareness Checklist and Screening Tools. J Am Diet Assoc 92: 163–67
80. White JV, Ham RJ, Lipschitz DA, Dwyer JT, Wellman NS (1991) Consensus of the Nutrition Screening Initiative: risk factors and indicators of poor nutritional status in older Americans. J Am Diet Assoc 91: 783–87
81. White House Conference on Aging (1981) Final Report of the 1981 White House Conference on Aging: A National Policy on Aging. Washington, DC: US Government Printing Office
82. World Bank (1993) World Development Report Investing in Health Oxford: Oxford University Press
83. Yasuda N, Zimmerman SI, Hawkes W, Fredman L, Hevel JR, Magaziner J (1997) Relation of social network characteristics to 5-year mortality among young-old versus old-old white women in an urban community. Am J Epidemiol 145: 516–23
84. Yates AA, Schlicker SA, Suiter CW (1998) Dietary reference intakes: the new basis for recommendations for calcium and related nutrients, B vitamins, and choline. J Am Dietet Assn 98: 699–706
85. Zandt SV, Fox H (1986) Nutritional impact of congregate meals programs. J Nutr Elderly 5: 31–43

Author's address:

Barbara E. Millen DPH, RD
Associate Dean for Research
Boston University School of Public Health
715 Albany Street
Boston, MA 02118, USA